POCKET DICTIONARY
Neurology Defined
Eponyms in Neurosciences

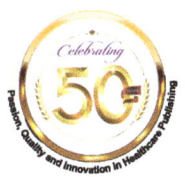

POCKET DICTIONARY

Neurology Defined
Eponyms in Neurosciences

Author

Kalyan B Bhattacharyya
MD DM MAMS FIAN FRCP (Edin)

Professor and Head
Department of Neurology
RG Kar Medical College and Hospital
Kolkata, West Bengal, India

Foreword

M Gourie Devi

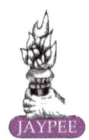

JAYPEE BROTHERS MEDICAL PUBLISHERS
The Health Sciences Publisher
New Delhi | London | Panama

Jaypee Brothers Medical Publishers (P) Ltd

Headquarters

Jaypee Brothers Medical Publishers (P) Ltd
4838/24, Ansari Road, Daryaganj
New Delhi 110 002, India
Phone: +91-11-43574357
Fax: +91-11-43574314
Email: jaypee@jaypeebrothers.com

Overseas Offices

J.P. Medical Ltd
83 Victoria Street, London
SW1H 0HW (UK)
Phone: +44 20 3170 8910
Fax: +44 (0)20 3008 6180
Email: info@jpmedpub.com

Jaypee-Highlights Medical Publishers Inc
City of Knowledge, Bld. 235, 2nd Floor, Clayton
Panama City, Panama
Phone: +1 507-301-0496
Fax: +1 507-301-0499
Email: cservice@jphmedical.com

Jaypee Brothers Medical Publishers (P) Ltd
Bhotahity, Kathmandu, Nepal
Phone: +977-9741283608
Email: kathmandu@jaypeebrothers.com

Website: www.jaypeebrothers.com
Website: www.jaypeedigital.com

© 2019, Jaypee Brothers Medical Publishers

The views and opinions expressed in this book are solely those of the original contributor(s)/author(s) and do not necessarily represent those of editor(s) of the book.

All rights reserved. No part of this publication may be reproduced, stored or transmitted in any form or by any means, electronic, mechanical, photocopying, recording or otherwise, without the prior permission in writing of the publishers.

All brand names and product names used in this book are trade names, service marks, trademarks or registered trademarks of their respective owners. The publisher is not associated with any product or vendor mentioned in this book.

Medical knowledge and practice change constantly. This book is designed to provide accurate, authoritative information about the subject matter in question. However, readers are advised to check the most current information available on procedures included and check information from the manufacturer of each product to be administered, to verify the recommended dose, formula, method and duration of administration, adverse effects and contraindications. It is the responsibility of the practitioner to take all appropriate safety precautions. Neither the publisher nor the author(s)/editor(s) assume any liability for any injury and/or damage to persons or property arising from or related to use of material in this book.

This book is sold on the understanding that the publisher is not engaged in providing professional medical services. If such advice or services are required, the services of a competent medical professional should be sought.

Every effort has been made where necessary to contact holders of copyright to obtain permission to reproduce copyright material. If any have been inadvertently overlooked, the publisher will be pleased to make the necessary arrangements at the first opportunity. The **CD/DVD-ROM** (if any) provided in the sealed envelope with this book is complimentary and free of cost. **Not meant for sale.**

Inquiries for bulk sales may be solicited at: jaypee@jaypeebrothers.com

Pocket Dictionary Neurology Defined: Eponyms in Neurosciences / Kalyan B Bhattacharyya

First Edition: 2019

ISBN: 978-93-5270-997-7

Printed at

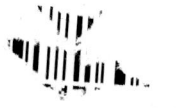

Dedication

Dedicated to my parents, my family, teachers, students and the neuroscientists, who with their tireless energy and endeavor, devoted their lives for the relief of the sufferings of countless number of hapless subjects.

Foreword

In an era with tremendous advances in clinical neurology along with related technologies which have led to precision in diagnosis and reduction in mortality and morbidity, it is of great interest that academic and practicing neurologists are interested in eponyms of neurological disorders. We continue to pay tribute to accomplished great masters and thinkers of antiquity and those of the immediate past and present era who had astute observation skills, meticulous documentation combined with reasoning and logical inference. Neurology an amalgam of art, skill and knowledge will continue to be a discipline which entails thorough and careful history taking and physical examination. In everyday clinical practice, the eponyms are frequently used and significance is immediately understood. Clinical symptoms and signs, wide range of neurological disorders, anatomical structures varying from gross to molecular level, physiological functions, pathological alterations, diagnostic and treatment modalities carry the names of the discoverers from few centuries ago extending forwards to the contemporary period.

It is a Herculean task to memorize the eponyms and recall them at the opportune and appropriate time, hence a dictionary of eponyms would be a valuable asset for ready reference. Professor Kalyan B Bhattacharyya has ventured to take the arduous task of compiling enormous number of eponyms with photographs and concise and succinct record of the salient observations. The interested clinician can easily navigate through the pages of the eponyms since they are listed alphabetically. This dictionary of eponyms is comprehensive, but not unwieldy and is eminently readable.

Professor Kalyan B Bhattacharyya is an eminent neurologist, outstanding teacher and researcher with special interest in movement disorders. His passion for history of neurology has in a great measure, enriched the book. The reader will be captivated by the eponyms and even the enlightened expert also enthralled by the contents. One is aware of the familiar Babinski phenomenon or sign, but may not be aware that there are at least five more eponyms including Babinski hammer. There are numerous similar examples which will fascinate the reader.

In summary, this encyclopedia provides a compendium of eponyms in neurology is a "must have" book that should be read by trainees, neurologists and other professionals allied to neurosciences.

M Gourie Devi
MD DM DSc FAMS FIAN FNASc
Chairperson
Department of Neurophysiology and
Senior Consultant Neurologist
Sir Ganga Ram Hospital
New Delhi, India

Preface

Medical literature teems with eponymous terms and one feels that perhaps in the field of neurosciences it is found in the most overwhelming manner. In a way, it is no wonder. The science pertaining to the nervous system evolved systematically by means of personal observations since the time of Hippocrates in the 4th century BC, Galen of Pergamon in the 2nd century, to Thomas Willis and Thomas Sydenham in the 17th century, and then, over the ages, by the contributions of Moritz Romberg, Jean Martin Charcot, Joseph Babinski, Jules Dejerine, Wilhelm Erb, Alois Alzheimer, Hughlings Jackson William Gowers, Gordon Holmes, Kinnier Wilson, PK Thomas, Ian McDonald, David Marsden, Anita Harding and others in the 19th and the 20th century. Investigations for neurological diseases were scarce and primitive, and the sharpest possible clinical acumen, along with the penchant for painstakingly pursuing their cherished goal by burning much midnight oil and candlesticks, were the only weapons in the armamentarium of these neuroscientists. It is therefore, quite natural that the diseases, signs, symptoms, syndromes, tests, and maneuvers they described have stood the ruthless grind of time and have been assured immortality. Indeed, it is well-nigh, impossible to expunge them from the medical vocabulary. No apposite and meaningful alternative term can yet to be conceived for Parkinson's disease, Huntington's disease, Wilson' disease, von Economo' disease, Romberg's sign, Tourette's syndrome, and the like.

I have attempted, within limitations, to arrange these eponymous conditions in an alphabetical order with a short description of the items and added photographs where possible. Many lesser known conditions, though of substantial import, have been left out since they are extremely rare and will only unnecessarily add to the bulk of the book. Owing to my incompetence in neurosurgical issues, I have intentionally desisted from dealing with esoteric surgical issues, like operative procedures and the like, and I hope some interested neurosurgeon shall take up the matter some day.

I am indebted to Professor Satish Khadilkar of Mumbai, and Dr Hrishikesh Kumar of Kolkata for kindly lending with some clinical photographs which I have incorporated in this volume.

Finally, I shall be amiss, if I fail to express my deepest gratitude and indebtedness to Professor M Gourie Devi, former Director and Vice Chancellor of National Institute of Mental Health and Neurosciences, and one of the most eminent neuroscientists from our country of international repute for kindly agreeing to write the foreword for this book. A scholar and researcher extraordinaire, I frequently communicated with her and most readily and unhesitatingly she enriched me with her apt and apposite comments in order to embellish the volume further. The erudite exposition in her foreword, written in chaste and elegant language, vividly reflects her perception about the subject.

Finally, I shall feel my job accomplished if the readers find the book readable and enjoyable.

Kalyan B Bhattacharyya

SECTION A

Abadie's sign There are two different signs associated with the name of Joseph Abadie of France.
- Loss of pain sensation on squeezing Achilles tendon in tabes dorsalis
- Spasm of levator palpebrae superioris muscle in thyrotoxicosis. This contributes partly to the wide palpebral fissure.

Achilles jerk The other name for ankle jerk.

Adamkiewicz artery It is the largest anterior segmental artery supplying the spinal cord. It typically arises from the left side from the abdominal aorta at the level of 9th to 12th intercostal artery and supplies the lower two-third of the spinal cord through the anterior spinal artery. Sometimes it arises from a lumbar vessel. Occlusion of this artery leads to motor weakness in the lower limbs along with urinary and fecal incontinence with preservation of posterior column functions, since the posterior part of the spinal cord is not supplied by this artery and therefore, spared.

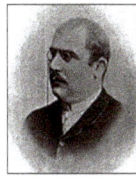

Albert Wojciech Adamkiewicz (1850–1921, Poland)

Adie's pupil Tonic pupil which dilates slowly in darkness and takes a long time to constrict in response to light. The accommodation reflex is normal. It is more commonly seen in women and when associated with absent knee or ankle jerk, it is known as *Holmes-Adie syndrome*, while concomitant impaired sweating in one side of the body is known as *Ross' syndrome*. The lesion lies in the ciliary ganglion, supplying postganglionic fibers of parasympathetic nerves to the iris following a viral infection. Abnormal sweating is consequent upon degeneration of the posterior root ganglion. Diagnosis is established by the observation of constriction of the pupil with low dose of pilocarpine, indicating denervation supersensitivity of Walter Cannon.

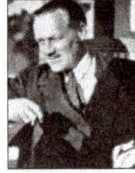

**William John Adie
(1886–1935, United Kingdom)**

Adie-Critchley syndrome
Forced grasping and groping reaction in tumor of the contralateral frontal lobe.

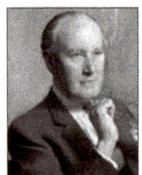

**Macdonald Critchley
(1900–1999, United Kingdom)**

Adrian's all-or-none law
The principle that the strength by which a nerve or muscle fiber responds to a stimulus is independent of the strength of the stimulus. If that stimulus exceeds the threshold potential, the nerve or muscle fiber will offer a complete response; otherwise, there is no response. It was first established by the American physiologist Henry Pickering Bowditch in 1871 for the contraction of heart muscle. However, it was proved experimentally by Edgar Adrian of Cambridge in 1928 which earned him the Nobel Prize in 1932.

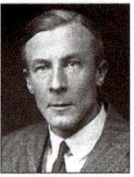

**Edgar Douglas Adrian
(1889–1977, United Kingdom)**

Adson's test A sign of thoracic outlet syndrome. The patient's arm is extended at the elbow and abducted and rotated posteriorly. There is loss of pulsation of the radial pulse when the patient rotates his head to the side tested and the examiner rotates and extends the patient's shoulder. The patient takes a deep breath and is asked to hold it and the test is considered positive if there is loss of radial pulse along with the appearance of radicular symptoms like, paresthesia. Sometimes, there is a bruit over the brachial artery. The hand may turn pale and is known as '*white hand sign*'. The test is no longer considered as that reliable, since many normal subjects show diminution of the radial pulse with this maneuver. *Roo's maneuver* is a related test, where the patient elevates and abducts his arms and identical symptoms are reproduced after 3 minutes.

Aicardi syndrome A constellation of agenesis of corpus callosum, infantile spasms and chorioretinal lacunae. Myoclonus, intellectual decline, microcephaly and optic nerve hypoplasia with morning glory appearance in the retina are additional features in some cases. The condition is seen exclusively in girls. It is an X-linked dominant condition at Xp22 locus and male fetuses die in utero. It has been described in boys with Klinefelter's syndrome.

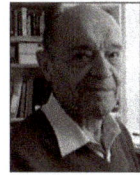

**Jean Aicardi
(1926–2015, France)**

Alexander's disease A fatal neurodegenerative condition in infants, characterized by developmental delay, enlarged head, seizures, spasticity, dementia and sometimes, idiopathic intracranial hypertension. There is mutation in the GFAP gene and the genetic defect in this autosomal dominant condition is in chromosome 17q21 position, though sporadic cases are commoner. Pathologically, megaencephaly is observed. It is a variety of leukodystrophy characterized by the presence of a variety of protein, *Rosenthal fibers*, in the astrocytes of the brain. Other causes of leukodystrophy with enlarged head include Canavan's disease and Van der Knapp's disease or megaencephalic leukodystrophy with subcortical cysts. In India, the latter condition has been described in the Agarwal community by Singhal and in a single Bengali girl by Bhattacharyya.

Alexander's law In spontaneous nystagmus due to unilateral vestibular lesion, the amplitude of the fast component increases when the subject looks towards the quick phase.

Alice in Wonderland syndrome It is a syndrome complex of micro- or macropsia, pelopsia (a feeling that subjects are nearer than they actually are), teleopsia (reverse of pelopsia), etc., and altered perception of body image. This is associated with migrainous aura or intake of psychotropic or psychedelic agents, like LSD. The name comes from the description of Lewis Carroll in Alice in Wonderland and it is believed that Carroll himself suffered from migraine.

Alpers' disease Also known as Alpers-Huttenlocher syndrome, it is a progressive neurodegenerative disorder of mitochondrial DNA depletion, characterized by delayed milestones, intractable seizures, particularly epilepsia partialis continua, myoclonus, areflexia, spasticity, dementia, optic atrophy and deafness. It is an autosomal recessive disorder occurring typically in childhood and is fatal. The disease can manifest as myopathic, encephalomyopathic, or hepatopathic patterns. The concerned genes are TK2 in myopathic, SUCL2 and RRM2B in encephalomyopathic, and DGUOK, POLG and MPV17 in hepatopathic variety.

Alport syndrome An oculorenal syndrome characterized by a triad of clinical findings consisting of hemorrhagic nephritis, sensorineural hearing loss and lenticonus, keratoconus, and cataracts. Diffuse leiomyomatosis and dissection of the aorta are occasionally observed. Most of the cases are of X-linked recessive inheritance with mutation in the COL4A3, COL4A4 and COL4A5 gene.

Alzheimer's baskets Condensed clumps of filaments between the nerve cells seen in advanced cases of Alzheimer's disease.

Alzheimer's cell type 1 Large multinucleated astrocytes found in glial tumor and progressive multifocal leukoencephalopathy.

Alzheimer's cell type 2 Swollen astrocytes with large nucleus and a significant nucleolus with little cytoplasm. They are metabolically active and found in cortex, brainstem, cerebellum and thalamus. They are classically found in hyperammonemic conditions like, hepatic encephalopathy, hepatocerebral degeneration and Wilson's disease.

Alzheimer's disease (The reader is referred to any standard textbook of neurology)

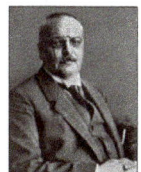

**Alois Alzheimer
(1864–1915, Germany)**

Alzheimer's sclerosis Degeneration of the middle and smaller cerebral blood vessels at a cellular level.

Alzheimer's stain A staining method for the detection of Negri bodies in rabies.

Anderson's disease The other name for glycogen storage disease type IV characterized by enzyme deficiencies affecting either glycogen synthesis, glycogen breakdown, or glycolysis, classically within the muscles. Of the various manifestations, the neuromuscular ones consist of late childhood development of myopathy and mild muscular weakness.

Angelman syndrome It is characterized by intellectual and motor developmental delay, microcephaly, speech and balance problem and seizures. The affected children are usually of an affable nature, hyperexcitable and they often flap their hands. They exhibit the tendency to handle water. The condition is caused by lack of function of the gene UBE3A, in chromosome 15, which is inherited from the mother. Sometimes, it is due to

Neurology Defined

inheritance of two copies of the chromosome from the father and none from the mother. *Prader–Willi syndrome* is a related condition where the disease is inherited from the father.

Anton syndrome Also known as *Anton–Babinski syndrome*, it is a condition where a blind person denies blindness and in order to prove their point, they tend to confabulate as if they can see. This happens with bilateral occipital infarction following posterior cerebral infarction, or as a complication of JC virus infection following the use of natalizumab in multiple sclerosis. It has also been described in rare cases of adrenoleukodystrophy, where both the occipital lobes undergo dysmyelination. Thus, it is a variety of visual anosognosia.

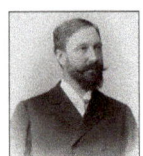

Gabriel Anton
(1858–1933, Austria)

Antoni A and B patterns In schwannoma, two varieties of cells are found in histological study. The fibrillary, polar and elongated tissue is known as *Antoni A pattern*, whereas the loose, less dense microcystic tissues in close proximity is known as *Antoni B pattern*. Antoni A is also known as *Verocay bodies*.

Apert syndrome A variety of acrocephalosyndactylism, where there is pronounced malformations in the bones in the skull, face, hands and feet, affecting the first branchial arch. Various malformations of the skull like, brachycephaly (the commonest variety, where the coronal and lambdoid sutures undergo fusion, leading to a transversely broad face and the parietal bones form the sides and the top of the head), trigonocephaly, dolicocephaly, plagiocephaly, turricephaly and oxycephaly have been described depending on the nature of fusion of cranial sutures in uterus. Syndactylism is a common accompaniment and the eyes protrude due to small orbit following premature fusion of the sutures between the frontal, sphenoid, zygomatic and maxillae. There is mutation in the FGFR2 gene which produces fibroblast growth factor and immature cells turn into osseous tissue. The condition is inherited as an autosomal dominant trait.

Aran-Duchenne disease The other name for amyotrophic lateral sclerosis.

Archimedes spiral This refers to drawing a spiral smoothly and elegantly from the center of the page to the periphery. In normal subjects it is well organized. However, in tremulous conditions, like in essential tremor or Parkinson's disease, it is clumsy and the gaps between the curves are irregular. In Parkinson's disease, the space between the lines is short, while the reverse is true for essential tremor.

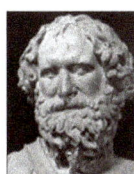

Archimedes of Syracuse (287–212 BC, Greece)

Argyll Robertson pupil A classic sign of neurosyphilis, particularly in tabes dorsalis. The pupils are small, eccentric, and irregular in the margin, reacts to accommodation but not to light reflex. The iris is brownish in color. The lesion is thought to be in the pretectal area of the midbrain and the Edinger–Westphal nucleus of the Warwick oculomotor nucleus complex. Syphilitic iritis producing local scarring is the possible etiology of the iris pathology. Other mesencephalic lesions like, diabetes mellitus with autonomic neuropathy, multiple sclerosis, Wernicke's encephalopathy, sarcoidosis, optic nerve disease, among other conditions, can also present with such a clinical condition and they have been assigned the name, *pseudo Argyll Robertson pupil*. A colorful name, *prostitute's pupil*, has also been assigned to it. *Reverse Argyll Robertson pupil*, where light reflex is normal but accommodation reflex is defective it is sometimes found in postencephalitic parkinsonism and Burkitt's lymphoma.

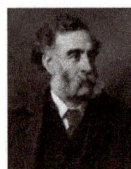

**Argyll Robertson
(1837–1909, United Kingdom)**

Arnold–Chiari malformations Structural defects in the cerebellum consisting of downward displacement of the cerebellar tonsils through the foramen magnum, sometimes causing non-communicating hydrocephalus. Classically, it is divided into four types, Type I, where there is tonsillar ectopia below the foramen magnum, sometimes with syringomyelia. The medulla and the brain stem may be elongated and kinked, while craniovertebral anomalies may be associated. Type II consists of displacement of the cerebellar vermis. It is sometimes associated with spina bifida and lumbar myelomeningocoele. Type III is associated with occipital encephalocoele, while Type IV is pure cerebellar hypo-

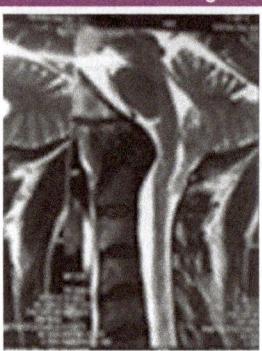

Figure A.1: Arnold–Chiari malformations. Note the descent of cerebellar tonsil below the foramen magnum

plasia, associated with Dandy–Walker syndrome. Cerebellar and pyramidal tract signs are the presenting features (Fig. A.1).

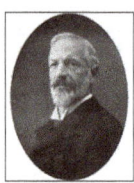

**Hans Chiari
(1851–1916, Austria)**

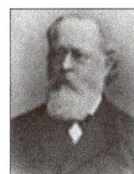

Julius Arnold
(1835–1915, Germany)

Ashworth scale A scale to assess the degree of spasticity. The grading runs from 0 or no spasticity to 4, when there is extreme spasticity in flexion or extension in ascending order of severity.

Asperger syndrome A disorder of development, it is characterized by difficulties in social interaction and nonverbal communication. Language is unaffected and intelligence is within normal limits. Some of them display stereotyped behavioral patterns like, preoccupation with one activity like stacking cans in a rack or arranging books for a long period of time, and the condition is often considered as a mild autism spectrum disorder. Flapping or twisting body movements or bending the whole body is a characteristic feature in some subjects. The speech is marked by limited prosody, tangentiality, circumstantiality and verbosity. Sometimes they can make socially inappropriate statements when strangers approach them, often known as verbal dysdecorum, or may yawn loudly during conversation. Some may show unusual hypersensitivity to sound, light and touch. Some have difficulty in falling asleep or maintaining it. No specific inheritance pattern is yet recognized.

Axenfeld-Schürenberg syndrome This is a congenital unilateral third cranial nerve palsy with mydriasis and alternate phases of pupillary constriction and contraction of muscles supplied by the oculomotor nerve. This leads to elevation of the upper lid and nasal deviation of the eye. This is autosomal dominant in inheritance and is also known as cyclic oculomotor palsy.

Avellis syndrome A variety of alternating paralysis involving the soft palate and the vocal cord

Avellis syndrome

of one side and hemianesthesia on the other side. It is usually the complication of occlusion of vertebral artery in lesions in the nucleus ambiguous and pyramidal tract in brain stem infarction. Sometimes, it is associated with Horner's syndrome with involvement of vagus and glossopharyngeal nerves.

SECTION B

Babcock sentence A sentence to assess memory. The patient is asked to remember the sentence '*One thing a nation must have to be rich and great is a large, secure supply of wood*'. The subject is asked to repeat it after 5 minutes. Normally, a subject is able to reproduce in 3 attempts.

Babinski hammer (Fig. B.1) Devised by Joseph Babinski in 1912, its handle is metallic and a round rubber is mounted on top of it. The handle is detachable.

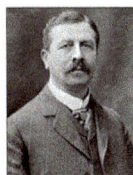

Joseph Jules François Félix Babinski (1857–1932, France)

Figure B.1: Babinski hammer

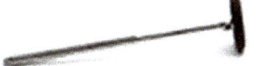

Babinski phenomenon A classic sign in neurology where in lesion of the corticospinal tract scratching the plantar aspect of the foot from the heel along the lateral aspect of the sole to just short of the ball of the great toe, results in extension of the great toe and fanning of the other toes. It is a component of mass reflex of Riddoch and was described in 1896.

Babinski sign II Diminished ankle jerk in sciatica.

Babinski Trunk-thigh test In organic hemiparesis, if the patient is asked to sit up with his arms folded over the chest, the paretic limb undergoes involuntary flexion. In hysterical hemiparesis, the normal limb will be flexed. In organic paraparesis, both the limbs shall move up and with a hysteric background, none shall move.

Babinski's the other sign In hemifacial spasm, when orbicularis oculi contracts to close the eyes, the ipsilateral frontal belly of occipitofrontalis contracts as well, as if in an attempt to open the contracting eye. Both the muscles are supplied by facial nerve and it is a tell-tale evidence that hemifacial spasm is an organic disorder. In any functional problem two antagonistic muscles cannot work in tandem.

Babinski–Fröhlich syndrome
The other name for dystrophia adiposogenitalis. It consists of obesity, hyperphagia, polyuria, polydypsia, hypogonadism and bitemporal hemianopia, resulting from pituitary adenoma or craniopharyngioma. It is caused by decreased level of gonadotropin-releasing hormone from the hypothalamus along with defect in the satiety center in the hypothalamus which leads to craving for food.

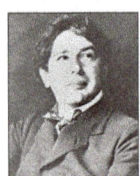

Alfred Fröhlich
(1871–1953, Austria)

Babinski–Nageotte syndrome
It is due to a paramedian pontine lesion leading to homolateral Horner's syndrome, weakness of soft palate, pharynx, larynx and tongue, loss of taste sensation in the posterior third of the tongue, cerebellar signs, with contralateral hemiparesis and hemianesthesia. The condition is very much like *Wallenberg's syndrome* or *Opalski syndrome*. However, in Wallenberg's syndrome, there is no hemiparesis since the corticospinal fibers are spared and in Opalski syndrome the lesion is more caudal and therefore, hemiparesis is in the ipsilateral side.

Babinski–Weil test When a patient complaining of vertigo, is asked to move ahead and back for ten steps each time in a straight line, he deviates to one side while moving forward and to the other side while coming back, as if walking in a star-shaped dimension.

Babkin reflex When the palm of a newborn baby is pressed, the mouth opens, neck is tilted back and the forearm is flexed. This normal reaction lasts up to the fourth month of life.

Baillarger lines Bands of fibers visible in sections of the cerebral cortex. Baillarger described six layers and these were confirmed later by Robert Remak of Prussia. The outermost band is most prominent in the occipital cortex which is known as the *band of Gennari*.

Baillarger sign This refers to unilateral dilatation of the pupil in tertiary syphilis.

Baillarger syndrome Also known as Frey's syndrome, it is a constellation of sweating in the cheek region, following gustatory stimulation, particularly after the intake of food items which leads to increased salivation like lemon. It is caused due to damage to the auriculotemporal nerve near the parotid glands, and it mostly follows surgical or traumatic insult, leading to aberrant regeneration of damaged parasympathetic fibers. Injection of botulinum toxin sometimes offers some relief.

Baillarger-Jackson principle It is the ability of subjects suffering from aphasia who cannot utter words at will, yet can enunciate involuntarily.

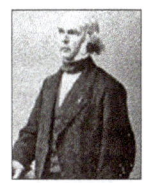

**Jules Baillarger
(1890–1900, France)**

Bálint syndrome The constellation of inability to perceive the visual field as a whole entity (simultagnosia), inability in reaching an object in the presence of normal visual acuity, (optic ataxia) and difficulty in fixating the eyes, (oculomotor apraxia). Usually, it has an acute onset due to ischemic insult in the borderzone area in the occipito-parietal region following severe hypotension. The condition is also known as *Bálint-Holmes syndrome*. Rarely, it can be the manifestation of a migrainous attack, traumatic brain injury, butterfly glioma, or Alzheimer's disease.

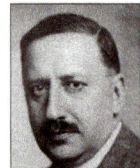

**Rezsö Bálint
(1874–1929, Hungary)**

Balo's concentric sclerosis

(Fig. B.2) This is a demyelinating condition and often considered a variant of multiple sclerosis, described by József Mátyás Baló from Hungary. The white matter classically shows alternate bands of demyelination and normal myelin, which looks like a transversely cut onion and are found in the frontal lobe. The onset is in childhood and spastic paraparesis is the classical presentation. The course is primary progressive, but relapsing-remitting variety is also known. Patients often respond to prednisolone therapy.

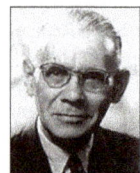

**József Mátyás Baló
(1895–1979, Hungary)**

Bárány's alarm apparatus A noise-producing apparatus that is placed in one ear to eliminate hearing while the other one is being examined.

Bárány's calorie test This refers to the development of nystagmus on irrigation of the external auditory meatus with hot and cold water. Hot water induces beating nystagmus to the same side, while cold water does the same to the other side. Absence or reduction of amplitude indicates labyrinthine disorder.

Bárány's chair test In this test, a person is seated in a chair which is rotated with the head of the subject placed 30° forward,

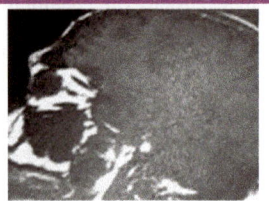

Figure B.2: Balo's Concentric sclerosis. Note the lower right quadrant of the photograph

which brings the horizontal semicircular canals in alignment with the horizontal plane. The subject wears an opaque spectacle or Frenzel's glasses in order to block ocular fixation. With normal labyrinthine function, horizontal nystagmus is seen with fast component to the direction of rotation. Its absence indicates vestibular pathology.

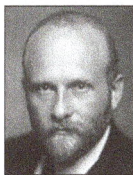

Robert Bárány
(1876–1936, Austria)

Bárány's past pointing test

A test for the integrity of the vestibular system, it utilizes the subject seated in a revolving chair with eyes closed which is rotated to the right for ten times. Thereafter, the subject holds his arm horizontally and the right index finger is brought to touch the examiner's finger and then the arm is raised vertically and again brings it in the horizontal position and repeats the maneuver. In cerebellar disease, the subject's finger will overshoot the examiner's finger to the side of the lesion, while in vestibular lesion, past pointing occurs with both the upper extremities towards the affected side.

Bárány's syndrome

A syndrome of unilateral headache in the back of the head with ipsilateral recurrent deafness, vertigo, tinnitus and abnormal pointing test and reduced irritability in Bárány's test.

Barnes' anterolateral tract

Some fibers of the corticospinal tract do not decussate at the medulla or upper spinal cord and descend ipsilaterally. They cross to the other side to synapse with the anterior horn cells thereafter at that spinal level. They constitute a very small percentage of the termination of the corticospinal tract. Thus, there are four ways the corticospinal tract synapses with the anterior horn cells. The huge majority of the fibers decussate at lower medulla and upper spinal cord and terminate in contralateral cells. Some fibers descend ipsilaterally to end at the same side. Some fibers cross to the other site and then again loop back to the same side. The other is *Barne's anterolateral tract* which crosses at the last moment to the opposite side.

Barré's sign The other name for pronator drift, a test to diagnose corticospinal tract lesion. When the upper limb is stretched in front with the palms turned up and the eyes closed, there is pronation, flexion of the elbow and a downward drift. The clinical importance of this test is that in mild hemiparesis, when muscle power may be normal, this sign may be positive.

Barthel index A scale of activities of daily living, in order to assess functional independence in a subject with neurological problems, especially, after cerebrovascular accident. The issues taken into consideration include, feeding, bathing, grooming, dressing, bowel control, bladder control, toileting, transfer from bed to chair and back, mobility on level surface and stairs.

Bassen-Kornzwig syndrome The other name for abetalipoproteinemia, where there is inability to absorb dietary fat through the intestine. It is autosomal recessive in inheritance where there is mutation in the microsomal triglyceride transfer protein resulting in deficiency in apolipoprotein B48 and B100. These are necessary for the synthesis and transport of VLDL and chylomicrons, respectively.

Batten's disease A fatal autosomal recessive disease of the nervous system in childhood, often known as neuronal ceroid lipofuscinoses (NCL), though most experts suggest that the term should be reserved for the NCL type 3. It is classified into infantile, late infantile, juvenile and adult form. Infantile form, the commonest variety, usually appears between 2 and 10 years of age and characterized by visual problems, seizures, behavioral problems, echolalia, and regression of milestones. At least 20 genes have been identified in association with Batten disease, while juvenile NCL, the most prevalent form of Batten's disease, has been linked to mutations in the CLN3 gene.

Battle's sign It refers to hematoma overlying the mastoid

Figure B.3: Racoon eye

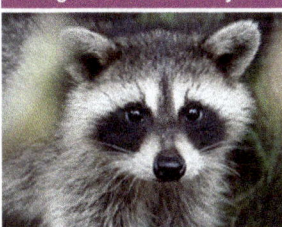

bone following head trauma, indicating underlying fracture of the base of the skull. It appears late, usually, 48–72 hours after the injury and it is stated to be a consistent sign of fracture of skull base. Sometimes it is associated with bilateral periorbital ecchymosis, when it is known as Racoon eye sign (Fig. B.3).

Becker's muscular dystrophy

A variety of X-linked recessive disorder characterized by slowly progressive muscular weakness. The onset is at around 8–10 years and there is weakness in the upper limbs and difficulty in walking. Gower's test is positive, where the subjects climbs over his legs and there is pseudohypertrophy of the calf muscles due to infiltration of fibrofatty tissue in the soleus and gastrocnemius. Cardiomyopathy is a common accompaniment as are various conduction defects. Sometimes there is scoliosis, muscle cramps, mental impairment and death is usually from pneumonia and respiratory failure. It is a variety of dystrophinopathy where dystrophin in skeletal muscles is less than normal. The diagnosis depends on high level of creatine kinase in blood, complex recruitment pattern on volition in electromyography, biopsy, and demonstration of lesser amount of dystrophin in muscles. Prognostically, it is better than *Duchenne muscular dystrophy*.

Becker's variety of myotonia congenita

The autosomal recessive variety of myotonia congenita where there is horizontal transmission of the disease in the families.

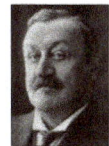

**Peter Emil Becker
(1908–2000, Germany)**

Neurology Defined

Beevor's sign Upward movement of the umbilicus in the supine position when the patient attempts to get up or flex his head over the chest against resistance applied by pressure by the examiner over the head. This indicates weakness of the abdominal muscles below the umbilicus and occurs with spinal cord lesion at the level of the T10 to T12 segment. This is also found positive in facioscapulohumeral muscular dystrophy.

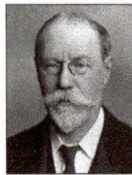

Charles Beevor
(1854–1908, United Kingdom)

Bejonet posture Hyperpronation and hyperflexion of the hands and feet with permanent dorsiflexion of the great toe, seen in advanced Parkinson's disease.

Bekhterev's sign In hemiplegia, if the upper limbs are abducted upto the level of the shoulder and asked to let them drop down, there is some perceptible delay in the downward movement in the affected limb. In hypotonic states the drop is more quick and abrupt.

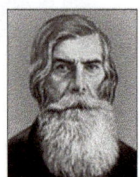

Vladimir Mikhailovich
Bekhterev (1857–1927, Russia)

Bell's nerve The other name for long thoracic nerve.

Bell's palsy Idiopathic lower motor neuron facial nerve palsy due to nonsuppurative infection of the facial nerve in the facial canal, usually following a viral infection. Factors indicating poor prognosis include, old age, diabetes mellitus, hypertension, lacrimation, hyperacusis, and limited recovery in 4 weeks time. Absence of blink reflex indicates poor prognosis and thus the study of blink reflex seems to be a useful index for predicting the prognosis in early stage of the paralysis.

Bell's phenomenon Reflex upward and mild outward movement of the eyeballs on closing the eyelids. This is the result of physiological synkinesis between the superior rectus and inferior oblique muscles of the eyeball. Though physiological, it cannot be recognized in a normal individual and is manifest in a case of Bell's palsy. This reflex indicates intact nuclear and infranuclear control of eye movement. However, some reports suggest that Bell's phenomenon may be absent in 10–15% of normal individuals. Though there is restriction of upgaze movement in Parinaud's syndrome, this reflex is sometimes preserved.

Bells' spasm Involuntary twitching of facial muscles.

Bell–Magendie law In spinal nerves the anterior root contains motor fibers and the posterior fibers contains sensory fibers and that nerve impulses are conducted in only one direction. Initially, Charles Bell from England said that the anterior root contains both motor and sensory fibers and the posterior root contains fibers from the cerebellum and autonomic fibers. This was corrected by François Magendie of France. The conjoint naming led to bitter acrimony between two of them which lasted till Bell's death.

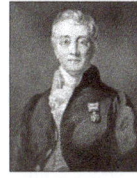

Charles Bell (1774–1842, United Kingdom)

Bender-Gestalt test A test of constructional ability, it is a dependable test for assessing paper and pencil drawing. The subject is presented with a series of simple and progressively more difficult line drawings, meant to be copied from memory. These are then assessed for errors of integration, distortion, perseveration and rotation.

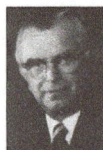

Morris Bender (1905–1983, United States of America)

Benedikt syndrome The constellation of oculomotor nerve palsy, ipsilateral cerebellar tremor and contralateral rubral tremor due a lesion in the region of the red nucleus and corticospinal tract.

Benedikt's inferior syndrome A pontine vascular lesion, causing contralateral hemiplegia, hemiataxia, and hemisensory loss.

Benton visual retention test A test for constructional ability, which evaluates reproduction, constructional ability, like design copying, and short term recall by utilizing construction from memory.

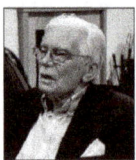

Arthur Lester Benton (1909–2006, United States of America)

Berger's waves The other name for the alpha waves in electroencephalography. This was the first electrocerebral wave identified by Hans Berger in Germany in 1929.

Bernhardt-Roth syndrome The other name for meralgia paresthetica.

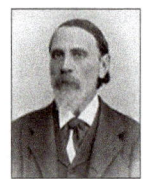

Moritz Benedikt (1835–1920, Austria)

Betz cells Also known as pyramidal cells of Betz, these are giant neurons in the fifth layer of grey matter in the primary motor cortex, or area 4 of Brodmann. These are the largest neurons in the central nervous system whose axons terminate as the corticospinal tract in the anterior horn cells of the spinal cord as wells as the nuclei of the bulbar muscles. However, corticospinal tract has its origin from cells other than the Betz cells.

Bickerstaff's encephalitis

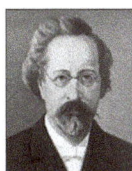

Vladimir Alekseyevich Betz
(1834–1894, Russia)

Bickerstaff's encephalitis A rare inflammatory condition of the brain, often affecting the peripheral nervous system as well. Ataxia and ophthalmoparesis are universal. Drowsiness, coma, hyper-reflexia, weakness of the limbs, face and bulbar muscles, pupillary abnormalities are the other features. It is usually a complication following lower respiratory tract infection and gastrointestinal upset. There is often overlap in the clinical features with Miller–Fisher syndrome and acute inflammatory demyelinating polyneuroradiculopathy and this raises the issue that this condition is an autoimmune disease. Anti-GQ1b antibody is positive in a large number of cases and cerebrospinal fluid analysis shows pleocytosis and elevated albumin level. Nerve conduction study reveals axonopathy and MRI scan shows scattered high intensity signals in T2-weighted image. The condition is treated with corticosteroids, plasmapheresis and intravenous immunoglobulin.

Bickerstaff's migraine

Bickerstaff's migraine Also known as *Bickerstaff syndrome* or vertebrobasilar migraine, it is a variety of migraine with aura. The common age of presentation is in childhood or adolescence and it affects males and females equally. Since it is caused by ischemia in the brain stem, signs and symptoms make it unmistakable. It presents with the usual symptoms of classical migraine and the additional features include teichopsia, prosopagnosia, fortification spectra, bilateral numbness in the lips, hands and feet, diplopia, dysarthria, ataxia, disorientation, vertigo, tinnitus, and loss of consciousness. Recovery is usually accompanied by occipital headache. With age basilar migraine is often replaced by migraine without aura. It is managed by NSAIDs and antiemetics like ondensetron or metoclopramide. Dietary restrictions, as advised for migraine are also of use.

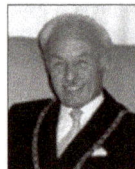

Edwin Robert Bickerstaff (1920–2007, United Kingdom)

Bielschowsky's disease The other name for early juvenile type of cerebral sphingolipidosis.

Bielschowsky's head tilt test In trochlear nerve palsy, the head is tilted towards the contralateral unaffected shoulder. The intorsion of the unaffected eye effected by the head tilt compensates for diplopia, caused by the 4th cranial nerve palsy.

Bielschowsky's squint Upward movement and inward rotation of the squinting eye as a sign of trochlear nerve paresis.

Biernacki's sign Absence of pain on pressing the ulnar nerve in tabes dorsalis.

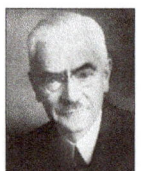

Alfred Bielschowsky (1869–1940, Germany)

Biot's breathing Strictly speaking this is not a neurological eponym, but this kind is breathing is often observed in a comatose subject. This is characterized by groups of quick, shallow inspirations followed by regular or irregular phases of apnea. It is caused by damage to the pons following stroke or road traffic accident due to uncal or tentorial herniation. Opiod abuse can also lead to this type of breathing.

Bjerrum's scotoma A comet-shaped area of loss of vision usually seen in glaucoma connected at the temporal side of the visual field to the blind spot or separated from it by a tiny gap.

Bjerrum's screen A flat black surface, used to measure the central 30 degrees of the visual field. The screen is made of black material and stitched with radial lines at 15 degree intervals and circles at 5 degree intervals.

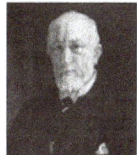

Jannik Petersen Bjerrum
(1851–1920, Denmark)

Bohan's diagnostic criterion

A criterion for diagnosis of dermatomyositis-polymyositis. It includes, symmetrical weakness of limb girdle muscles and anterior neck flexors, muscle biopsy showing evidence of characteristic myositis, elevated serum skeletal muscle specific enzyme, particularly creatine phosphokinase, electromyographic evidence of myositis, and typical dermatomyositis rash, including *Gottron's papule*.

Bonnet phenomenon A modification of straight leg raising test where the thigh and leg are adducted and internally rotated.

Bourneville's disease (Fig. B.4) The other name for tuberous sclerosis. It is characterized by epilepsy, low intelligence and adenoma sebaceum, and hence

Figure B.4: Bourneville's disease, showing profuse adenoma sebaceum. CT scan shows subependymal tubers

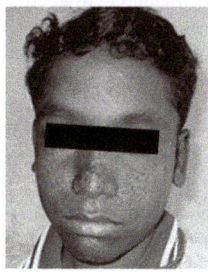 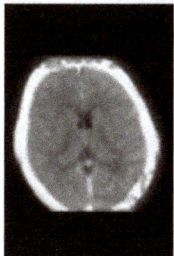 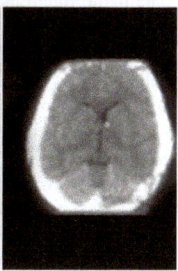

the acronym, epiloia. The last entity is a misnomer since they are actually fibromas. Other features include shagreen patch and salmon patch at the back, subungual fibromas, renal angioma which may bleed and lead to hematuria and rhabdomyosarcoma of the heart. In the eyes, retinal hamartomas or phakomas are observed. Ash leaf macules can be seen at the back with the help of Wood's lamp which utilizes ultraviolet rays. Actually, the first patient described by Bourneville suffered from rhabdomyosarcoma of the heart. Since there are so many diverse clinical features, the condition is now known as *tuberous sclerosis complex*.

The name tuberous sclerosis is derived from the presence of thick nodular gyri in the brain, called tubers. It is an autosomal dominant disease with incomplete penetrance, though sporadic mutations are more common. It is linked to two genetic loci TSC1 and TSC2. The former codes for the protein, hamartin, and is located on chromosome 9q34, whereas the latter codes for the protein, tuberin and is on chromosome 16p13.3.

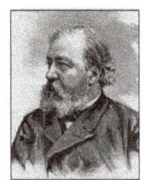

Désiré-Magloire Bourneville (1840–1909, France)

Bourneville-Brissaud disease The other name for tuberous sclerosis. Incidentally, Brissaud studied one of the earliest diagnosed cases with Désiré Magloire Bourneville, the neuroscientist who described the condition and whose first patient died of rhabdomyosarcoma of the heart.

Bragard's sign A modification of straight leg raising test where the foot is passively dorsiflexed also.

Briquet syndrome The other name for somatization disorder characterized by recurring, multiple somatic symptoms in the absence of any definite clinically elicitable sign.

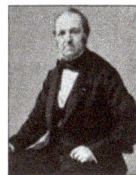

**Pierre Briquet
(1796–1881, France)**

Brissaud reflex A sign for corticospinal tract disorder where scratching the lateral aspect of the sole leads to contraction of the ipsilateral tensor fascia lata.

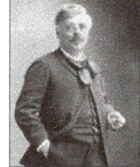

**Édouard Brissaud
(1852–1909, France)**

Brissaud's disease The other name for Tourette syndrome.

Brissaud-Sicard syndrome Hemiparesis and contralateral hemifacial spasm resulting from a pontine lesion.

Broca's aphasia Also known as anterior, nonfluent, expressive, or motor aphasia, this is caused by a lesion in the third frontal convolution of the inferior frontal lobule in the dominant hemisphere. The usual etiology is a vascular pathology. The prominent features are telegraphic speech with preserved comprehension and impaired repetition. Naming is also impaired and alexia and agraphia can be other features. Sometimes this variety of aphasia is seen during recovery from global aphasia.

Broca's area It lies in the inferior frontal convolution just anterior to the face area of the motor cortex and above the Sylvian fissure in the dominant, usually left side. This is also known as area 44 of Brodmann. Lesion in this area leads to expressive dysphasia, also known as anterior, nonfluent, or motor dysphasia. The subject in whom the French surgeon Paul Broca described the lesion, could utter only one work, Tan. He was therefore, referred to as *Tan*. Autopsy revealed a syphilitic lesion. However, Broca was challenged by Pierre Marie who even dug up the grave and it was seen that the lesion was actually in the parieto-occipital region.

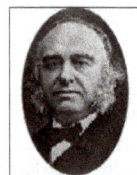

Pierre Paul Broca (1824–1880, France)

Brodmann's area Areas in the cerebral cortex which are arbitrarily numbered based on cytoarchitectural differences and cellular organization in different anatomical regions. There are 52 such areas and the well known ones include areas 1, 2, 3 for sensory cortex, 4 for motor cortex, 6 for premotor cortex 17 for primary visual cortex, 18, 19 for visual association cortex, 41, 42 for primary auditory cortex, 44 for speech control, or Broca's area, etc.

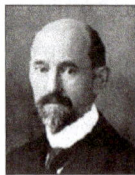

Korbinian Brodmann (1868–1918, Germany)

Brown syndrome Also known as superior tendon sheath syndrome, it is a rare congenital or acquired disorder where there is restriction in elevation of the eye, particularly in the adducted position. It is caused by malfunction of the superior oblique muscle, like shortening or tightening of the superior oblique tendon, while it hooks round the trochlea in the frontal bone.

Brown-Séquard syndrome This classic condition is seen in hemisection of the spinal cord where there is ipsilateral spasticity and weakness below the level of the lesion due to involvement of the corticospinal tract and segmental lower motor neuron signs at the level of the lesion due to anterior horn cell involvement. On the contralateral side, the findings are loss of pain and temperature sensation, as well as fine touch and vibration, below the lesion due to damage to the crossing lateral spinothalamic tract and posterior column respectively. This was a frequently seen morbidity due to bullet or stab injury in war times.

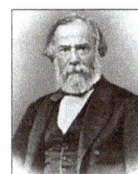

Charles-Edouard Brown-Séquard (1817–1894, Mauritius)

Brownell-Oppenheimer variant Creutzfeldt-Jakob disease A purely cerebellar presentation with progressive unsteadiness and incoordination which progresses for several weeks before the appearance of other features.

Brudzinski's sign In meningeal irritation due to meningitis or subarachnoid hemorrhage, passive flexion of the neck over chest leads to flexion of the thighs and legs. This is often known as *Brudzinski's sign I*. The *sign II* is elicited by flexing one thigh over abdomen and the leg over the thigh. In both the tests the patient complains of pain due to stretching and irritation of the spinal nerves from the inflamed meninges. There are two other less performed clinical tests in the name of Brudzinski, namely *cheek sign* and *Symphyseal sign*, where pressure over the cheek and symphysis pubis respectively, elicits flexion response in the lower limbs in meningitis.

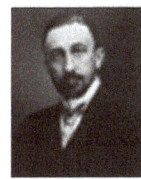

Joséf Brudziński (1874–1917, Poland)

Brueghel syndrome This is identical with Meige's syndrome, a combination of blepharospasm and oromandibular dystonia.

Bruns apraxia The tendency to fall back in bilateral lesions of the frontal lobe, like in cerebrovascular accident. Normal pressure hydrocephalus is another common condition. The pathology lies in the frontopontocerebellar tract which connects the frontal lobe to the cerebellum. There is start hesitation while walking with normal power and coordination in the lower limbs. The gait is broad-based with short steps. Other features include poor truncal mobility, falls following minimal postural disturbance, magnetic gait where there is inability to raise the feet from the floor, and turning en bloc, which is often known as the *pivot sign*. The subjects often reveal frontal lobe release signs and urinary incontinence.

Bruns nystagmus Combination of cerebellar and vestibular nystagmus found in lesions in the cerebellopontine angle, particularly acoustic schwannoma. Both the vestibular division of the 8th cranial nerve and cerebellar peduncles are involved in these lesions. It is characterized by slow, large amplitude gaze paretic nystagmus while looking towards the side of the lesion and rapid small amplitude vestibular nystagmus while to the other side.

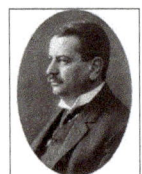

Ludwig Bruns
(1858–1915, Germany)

Brushfield's spots Small grayish spots of depigmentation in the iris in Down's syndrome.

Buchem syndrome Also known as hyperostosis corticalis generalisata it is a rare hereditary disorder where there is progressive sclerosing dysplasia of the diaphysis of long bones, mandible, clavicles and ribs. THRA1 gene is often implicated in its genesis and genomic deletion on chromosome 17q12-q21 is the feature. It closely resembles osteopetrosis.

Bumke's pupil Dilatation of the pupil in anxiety which fails to respond to light and accommodation.

Bunina bodies Small eosinophilic neuronal inclusion bodies in the bulbar or anterior horn cells in amyotrophic lateral sclerosis. It is considered a pathological hallmark of the disease. They are also found occasionally in the large X cells in the anterolateral aspect of the sacral nuclei, supplying the urinary bladder via nervi erigentes, though bladder involvement is classically absent in this condition. They contain two proteins, cystatin C and transferrin. The precise mechanism of its formation is not yet known.

Burdach column The other name for fasciculus cuneatus, carrying proprioceptive fibers from the upper limb and the upper half of the trunk in the posterior column, lying medial to the tract of Goll.

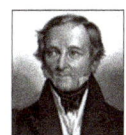

Karl Friedrich Burdach (1776–1847, Germany)

Buzzard reflex A variant of the knee jerk where the patient sits and presses on the floor as a facilitatory procedure.

SECTION C

Cajal cells These are interstitial cells in the intestinal wall. Myenteric interstitial cells serve as pacemaker which leads to coordinated muscular contraction.

Cajal nucleus A group of medium-sized neurons in the dorsomedial part of the mesencephalic tegmentum, lateral to nucleus of Darkschewitsch and together they receive fibers from the vestibular nuclei through the medial longitudinal fasciculus. Thereafter, they send fibers to the oculomotor nuclei via the posterior commissure. These nuclei and their connections integrate the movements of the head and the eye in vertical and oblique gaze.

Cajal stain A silver stain devised by Camillo Golgi from Italy and perfected by Ramón y Cajal from Spain. Cajal unearthed many facts about the structure of the nervous system in the process and the concept of neuron doctrine was thus born. They were jointly awarded the Nobel Prize in 1906.

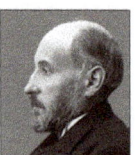

Santiago Ramón y Cajal (1852–1934, Spain)

Cajal's neural doctrine The doctrine has three components. Firstly, nerve cells are independent elements that do not anastomose, like in a syncytium, as his great contemporary, Camillo Golgi proposed, but make connections only at specific points. Secondly, nervous impulses are always transmitted from the cell body out to the axon and thirdly, the axon conducts away from the cell body. This led him to formulate the *law of dynamic polarization* which states that information runs in one direction through a neuron, from the dendrites, through the cell body, to the axon.

Canavan's disease A variety of leukodystrophy in early

infancy, characterized by growth retardation, hypotonia, megaencephaly and seizures. It is an autosomal recessive disorder with defect in the ASPA gene.

Cannon's law Also known as the law of denervation, it states that when efferent neurons are destroyed, there is an increased susceptibility of responding to the chemical substance it produces normally, the effect being maximal in the part denervated.

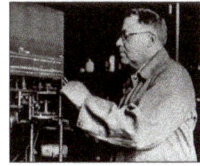

Walter Bradford Cannon
(1871–1945, United States of America)

Capgras syndrome Delusional syndrome encountered in psychiatric practice where the patient can recognize a member of the family or a close friend but believes that the subject has been replaced by an identical individual. Thus, it is a duplication phenomenon. It is seen in psychiatric conditions, Alzheimer's disease, traumatic brain injury and chronic metabolic disorders, like diabetes mellitus. Some authorities feel that it is a variety of Geschwind's disconnection syndrome where the visual recognition pathway is disconnected from the limbic system, where faces can be recognized but no emotional content is attached to it.

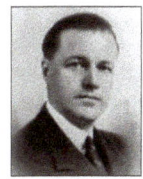

Joseph Capgras
(1873–1950, France)

Caplan's top of basilar artery syndrome Infarction of the rostral brainstem and hemisphere supplied by the distal basilar artery leads to visual, oculomotor and behavioral problems, with or without motor paralysis. Excessive sleepiness, hallucinations and dreamy behavior may be the other accompaniments. Usually it is caused by an embolic stroke.

It was first described by Louis Caplan of USA in 1980.

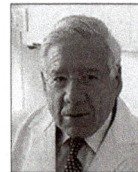

Louis Caplan (1936–till date, United States of America)

Chaddock's sign A sign of corticospinal tract damage where the upgoing great toe is elicited by scratching the skin below the lateral malleolus of the fibula in a circular manner from just above the lateral malleolus downwards. This sign is often positive for longer time than Babinski sign and may be found positive bilaterally in unilateral lesion.

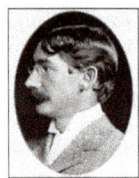

Charles Gilbert Chaddock (1861–1936, United States of America)

Chamberlain line An imaginary line joining the back of the hard palate to the posterior lip of the foramen magnum in the lateral view of the skull. If the odontoid process of the second cervical vertebra in 3 mm or more above this line, basilar invagination is present.

Charcot artery Other name for lenticulostriate artery, a branch of the M1 segment of the middle cerebral artery, which enters the base of the brain through the anterior perforated substances and supplies the striatum, globus pallidus and internal capsule. Rupture leads to massive hemorrhage.

Charcot disease The other name for amyotrophic lateral sclerosis.

Charcot joint A destructive arthropathy in big joints following repetitive trauma in conditions like syringomyelia, hereditary sensory motor neuropathy, neurosyphilis, leprosy, diabetic neuropathy, etc. It is usually, a painless condition.

Charcot laryngeal vertigo The other name for cough syncope where a subject becomes unconscious following a bout of violent cough. This is due to the operation of Valsalva mechanism, obstruction to ventricular filling and the subsequent reduced distribution of blood to the brain through the left ventricle and the carotid artery.

Charcot sign Elevation of the eyebrow on the side of a lower motor facial palsy and its depression when the patient attempts to close the eyelids.

Charcot triad The constellation of intention tremor, nystagmus and scanning speech found in multiple sclerosis due to involvement of the brainstem.

Charcot–Bouchard aneurysm Also known as miliary aneurysm, these refer to the small aneurysmal dilatation of less than 300 micrometer capillaries in the branches of lenticulostriate arteries which supply the basal ganglia. These are associated with chronic hypertension and are prone to rupture. This constituted the doctoral thesis for Charles Joseph Bouchard and the priority of names led to his bitter acrimony with his mentor, Jean Martin Charcot, leading finally to the failure of Joseph Felix Francois Babinski for the post of *Professor Agrégé* in 1892 where Bouchard was the examiner.

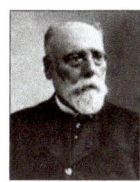

Charles Joseph Bouchard (1837–1915, France)

Charcot-Erb paresis The other name for syphilitic myelitis.

Charcot-Joffroy syndrome The other name for hypertrophic spinal meningitis.

Charcot–Marie–Tooth disease The previous name for hereditary sensory motor neuropathy which was also known as peroneal muscular atrophy. Usually the initial symptom is foot drop or hammer toe and wasting of the lower part of the lower limbs, giving the leg what is known as '*inverted champagne bottle appearance*'. Often there is pes cavus, scoliosis and neuropathic pain. The commonest cause is duplication of the short arm of chromosome 17 due to mutation in the PMP22 gene. It is divided into CMT1, CMT3 and CMT4 of demyelinating varieties and CMT2, which is of axonal type. Most cases are inherited in an autosomal dominant manner, though recessive transmission is sometimes observed in CMT4, and a few CMT2 subtypes. Diagnosis is established by nerve conduction study which shows prolongation of the latency in demyelinating variety and reduction of amplitude in the axonal type. The delayed latency is uniform in all nerves and thus differs from that of acquired demyelination. Nerve biopsy shows characteristic '*onion bulb appearance*' due to repeated demyelination and remyelination.

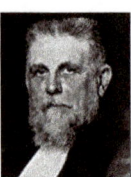

Pierre Marie
(1853–1940, France)

Charcot–Wilbrand syndrome

Visual agnosia and the inability to reconstruct visual image due to occlusion of the posterior cerebral artery of the dominant side.

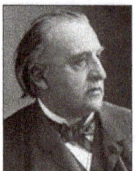

Jean Martin Charcot
(1825–1893, France)

Charles Bonnet syndrome

This refers to well-formed visual hallucinations in incompletely blind elderly persons, who can realize the problem and therefore the term '*pseudohallucination*' is preferred. The visual problems include bilateral cataracts, macular degeneration, and glaucoma. It is postulated that reduced visual acuity leads to hyperexitablity in the visual cortex. This is commonly seen with both the eyes closed.

Chaudhuri–Trenkwalder sleep scale

(Fig. C.1) A new sleep scale to quantify various aspects of nocturnal sleep problems in Parkinson's disease, which affects up to 96% of subjects.

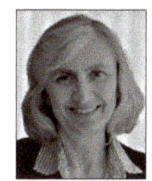

Claudia Trenkwalder (United States of America)

Cheyne–Stokes breathing

Strictly speaking this is not a neurological eponym, but this kind of breathing is often observed in a

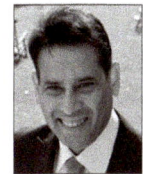

K Ray Chaudhuri (1958–till date, United Kingdom)

Figure C.1: Chaudhuri–Trenkwalder sleep scale

Please rate the severity of the following based on your experiences during the past week (7 days). Please make a cross in the answer box

	Very often (This means 6 to 7 days a week)	Often (This means 4 to 5 days a week)	Sometimes (This means 2 to 3 days a week)	Occasionally (This means 1 day a week)	Never
1. Overall, did you sleep well during the last week?	☐ 0	☐ 1	☐ 2	☐ 3	☐ 4
2. Did you have difficulty falling asleep each night?	☐ 4	☐ 3	☐ 2	☐ 1	☐ 0
3. Did you have difficulty staying asleep?	☐ 4	☐ 3	☐ 2	☐ 1	☐ 0
4. Did you have restlessness of legs or arms at nights causing disruption of sleep?	☐ 4	☐ 3	☐ 2	☐ 1	☐ 0
5. Was your sleep disturbed due to an urge to move your legs or arms?	☐ 4	☐ 3	☐ 2	☐ 1	☐ 0

Continued

Continued

Please rate the severity of the following based on your experiences during the past week (7 days). Please make a cross in the answer box					
	Very often (This means 6 to 7 days a week)	Often (This means 4 to 5 days a week)	Sometimes (This means 2 to 3 days a week)	Occasionally (This means 1 day a week)	Never
6. Did you suffer from distressing dreams at night?	☐ 4	☐ 3	☐ 2	☐ 1	☐ 0
7. Did you suffer from distressing hallucinations at night (seeing or hearing things that you are told do not exist)?	☐ 4	☐ 3	☐ 2	☐ 1	☐ 0
8. Did you get up at night to pass urine?	☐ 4	☐ 3	☐ 2	☐ 1	☐ 0
9. Did you feel uncomfortable at night because you were unable to turn around in bed or move due to immobility?	☐ 4	☐ 3	☐ 2	☐ 1	☐ 0
10. Did you feel pain in your arms or legs which woke you up from sleep at night?	☐ 4	☐ 3	☐ 2	☐ 1	☐ 0
11. Did you have muscle cramps in your arms or legs which woke you up whilst sleeping at night?	☐ 4	☐ 3	☐ 2	☐ 1	☐ 0
12. Did you wake early in the morning with painful posturing of arms and legs?	☐ 4	☐ 3	☐ 2	☐ 1	☐ 0
13. On waking, did you experience tremor?	☐ 4	☐ 3	☐ 2	☐ 1	☐ 0
14. Did you feel tired and sleepy after waking in the morning?	☐ 4	☐ 3	☐ 2	☐ 1	☐ 0
15. Did you wake up at night due to snoring or difficulties with breathing?	☐ 4	☐ 3	☐ 2	☐ 1	☐ 0

comatose subject. It is a variety of periodic breathing, characterized by progressively deeper and sometimes, faster breathing, followed by decrease with resultant apnea and followed by repeat, each episode lasting for 30 seconds to 2 minutes. It happens in damage to the respiratory center and the causes include congestive cardiac failure, renal failure, raised intracranial tension, narcotic poisoning, brain trauma, metabolic encephalopathies and brain tumors.

Chvostek's sign In hypocalcemia, tapping the facial nerve on exit from the stylomastoid foramen leads to twitching of the facial muscles. Possibly it is caused by higher discharge from the central pathway.

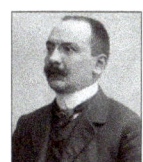

František Chvostek (1835–1884, Czechoslovakia)

Clapham's sign In damage to the facial nerve, there is contraction of the facial muscles on mechanical stretching of the cheek. This indicates preserved activity in the excitation and contraction mechanism of the facial muscles.

Claude Bernard's syndrome Ipsilateral pupillary dilatation, eyelid lag, diminished blinking, and increased lacrimation.

Claude's syndrome Ipsilateral oculomotor palsy with contralateral ataxia and choreiform movement due to lesion in the red nucleus.

Cogan's eyelid twitch sign In myasthenia gravis, if the eyes are moved from downgaze position to the primary position, there is a transient contraction in the upper eyelid by levator palpebrae superioris. This is followed by elevation of the globe caused by the contraction of the superior rectus muscle. It is caused by differential weakness of the two muscles and can also be seen in Miller-Fisher syndrome.

Cogan's oculomotor apraxia A rare congenital disorder characterized by defect in horizontal eye movements. Affected children fail to fixate on a target, the eyes lag behind and move in the opposite direction. They jerk their head past the object in an effort to bring the eyes in contact with the object. It is inherited as an autosomal recessive trait.

Cogan's rule In asymmetric optokinetic nystagmus the lesion is likely to be in the parietal lobe and not of vascular origin.

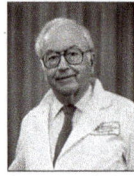

David Glendenning Cogan
(1908–1993, United States of America)

Collet-Sicard syndrome Paralysis of the 9th, 10th, 11th and 12th cranial nerve due to fracture of the base of the posterior fossa.

Collier's false localizing sign Paralysis of the abducent nerve in pathological conditions, where there is no lesion in the nerve proper. In certain conditions, the nerve is jeopardized in its long intracranial course and lesions elsewhere may lead to herniation of the lower brain stem. This results in bowing of the abducent nerve across structures, like the petrosphenoid ligament joining the apex of the petrous part of the temporal bone and the greater wing of the sphenoid bone. This hooking of the nerve leads to temporary abolition of the functions of the concerned nerve, and one is often led to believe that it is the 6th cranial nerve which is involved in the pathological process.

Collier's sign This refers to the elevation and retraction of the upper eyelids when the eyes are in primary position or in upward gaze. This is seen in conditions involving the upper dorsal midbrain supranuclear connections like, Parinaud's syndrome, top of the basilar syndrome, etc.

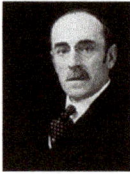

James Collier
(1870–1935, United Kingdom)

Corti's organ The receptor in the cochlea in the inner ear containing hair cells which respond to vibrations following movement of the cochlear fluid.

Costen syndrome The other name for temporomandibular joint arthritis characterized by pain during mastication or on movement of the lower jaw.

Cotard's syndrome Classical delusional syndrome where a subject denies his/her existence and believes that he/she is long dead. This is found in schizophrenia, severe depression, organic damage to non-dominant temporoparietal region, migrainous aura, etc.

Creutzfeldt–Jakob disease A fatal prion disease of the brain occurring mostly sporadically or inherited in an autosomal dominant manner, or sometimes acquired through contamination in an iatrogenic manner like, in corneal transplant, pituitary hormone therapy, blood transfusion and sperm donation. Variant disease is acquired from bovine spongiform encephalopathy after consumption of beef. This is also known as *Mad Cow Disease*. Clinically, it presents as rapidly progressive dementia and myoclonic jerks. Two varieties are recognized like, *Heidenhain variant* with prominent visual malfunctioning due to lesion in the occipital lobe and the *Brownell-Oppenheimer variant* with prominent cerebellar features like, ataxia. The electroencephalogram is characteristic with short duration burst-suppression pattern or triphasic waves. Cerebrospinal fluid shows the presence of 14-3-3 protein and the MRI shows characteristic cortical ribbon sign, pulvinar hyperintensity, and the hockey stick sign in the globus pallidus.

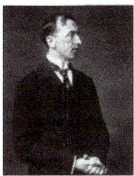

Hans Gerhard Creutzfeldt (1885–1964, Germany)

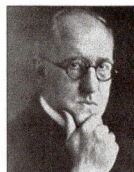

**Alfons Maria Jakob
(1885–1931, Germany)**

Crichton-Browne sign Tremulousness in the outer corner of the mouth and lips in general paralysis of the insane. James Crichton-Browne, is however, more famed for being one of the founding editors of the journal Brain 1877, along with Hughlings Jackson, David Ferrier and John Bucknill.

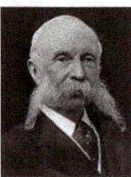

**James Crichton-Browne
(1840–1938, United Kingdom)**

Crouzon's disease (Fig. C.2) Autosomal dominant craniosynostosis with hypertelorism. The head shape is abnormal and the eyes protrude out of the socket with growth. There is premature closure of the sutures, particularly the sagittal and the coronal ones. Mutation in the fibroblast growth factor receptor II in chromosome 10 is the cause and the transmission is autosomal dominant in nature. Associated conditions are patent ductus arteriosus, coarctation of the aorta, short humerus and femur. The CT scan shows chronic compensated hydrocephalus.

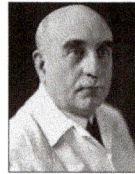

**Octave Crouzon
(1874–1938, France)**

Crowe's sign Axillary freckles in neurofibromatosis type I, found in about 30% cases and is considered one of the seven diagnostic criteria for the disease. These freckles may also be seen in inguinal region, nape of the neck and submammary areas.

Figure C.2: Crouzon's disease

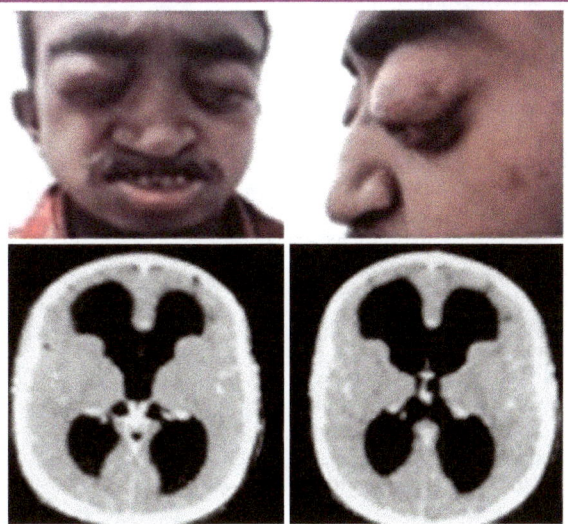

The other Crowe's sign refers to lateral sinus thrombosis when compression of the jugular vein in the normal side causes engorgement of retinal vessels.

Cushing syndrome A combination of signs caused by hypercortisolemia. These include hypertension, truncal obesity, thin limbs, buffalo hump, moon face, muscular wasting and weakness, osteoporosis, acne and reddish striae over abdomen. Headaches and depression are common accompaniments.

Cushing's disease When Cushing's syndrome is caused by excessive secretion of adrenocorticotrophic hormone from the anterior pituitary, it is called Cushing's disease. This is caused either by pituitary basophilic adenoma or due to excessive production of hypothalamic corticotrophin releasing hormone.

Cushing's law An acute increase of intracranial pressure also causes compression of the cerebral blood vessels and cerebral ischemia, producing an increase of systemic blood pressure, with simultaneous reduction in heart rate, and respiratory slowing.

Cushing's reflex A constellation of increased systolic blood pressure, pulse pressure, bradycardia, and slow irregular respiration in increased intracranial tension. This is usually seen in lesions in the posterior fossa like a tumor or massive hemorrhage and is indicative of impending herniation through the foramen magnum.

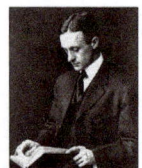

Harvey William Cushing (1869–1939, United States of America)

Cushing-Bailey's syndrome A syndrome of unsteadiness, disturbed coordination of the body in space, though with good coordination when lying or with body well braced.

Cushing-Rokitansky ulcer Gastrointestinal hemorrhage, complicating head injury.

Czarnecki's sign This is a synkinetic syndrome where due to aberrant regeneration of the oculomotor nerve to the sphincter of the iris, there is gaze-evoked segmental iris contraction. This is usually seen with the slit lamp.

SECTION D

Dagnini sign In pyramidal tract lesion tapping the radial aspect of the dorsum of the hand leads to extension of the wrist.

Dale principle One neuron uses only one neurotransmitter in all the terminals. This concept has been criticized in recent times.

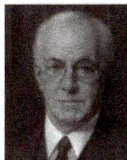

**Henry Hallett Dale
(1875–1968, United Kingdom)**

Dalrymple's sign Increased breadth of the palpebral fissure in hyperthyroidism.

Dandy's operation Retroganglial neurotomy for surgical therapy in trigeminal neuralgia.

Dandy's phenomenon A peculiar form of mock movement seen in loss of labyrinthine senses following bilateral damage to the vestibular nerves.

Dandy-Walker syndrome The commonest posterior fossa malformation in children characterized by the triad of cerebellar vermis hypoplasia and its cephalad rotation, dilatation of the fourth ventricle and its posterior extension, and abnormally high tentorium with the torcula placed above the level of the lambdoid. When the classical criteria is not met, they are known as Dandy-Walker variant or Dandy-Walker complex, which is of lesser clinical severity. It is considered a variant of ciliopathy.

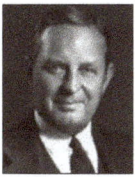

**Walter Edward Dandy
(1886–1946, United States of America)**

Darkschewitsch nucleus The nucleus of the posterior commissure within the third ventricle, anterior to Edinger-Westphal nucleus.

Daur-Babinski sign Tonic dorsiflexion of the great toe in Parkinson's disease or other related disorders of the basal ganglia. This is somewhat like the more commonly known condition, the *striatal toe* or *dystonic* toe, first recognized by Purves-Stewart in the National Hospital, Queen Square in 1906, while he had been working as a house physician.

Dawson's fingers Perpendicular demyelinating plaques on the corpus callosum in multiple sclerosis, as seen in sagittal T2-weighted MRI scan (Fig. D.1).

Figure D.1: Dawson's fingers

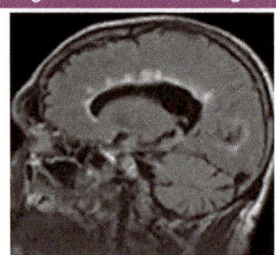

De Barsy syndrome A congenital disorder characterized by dysmorphic features cutis laxa, cloudy cornea, short stature, sparse hair, premature aging, delayed closure of fontanelle, cutis laxa, involuntary movements and developmental delay (Fig. D.2).

Figure D.2: De Barsy syndrome. Note dysmorphic features, cutis laxa

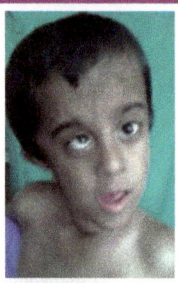

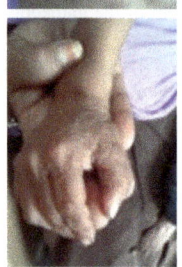

de Lange syndrome A dysmorphic syndrome characterized by growth retardation, diminished stature, mental retardation, palpebral fissures resembling Treacher-Collins syndrome where the outer canthus of the eye is at a lower level than the inner one, flexion contractures of elbows, clinodactyly, transverse palmar crease etc.

Deiters' nucleus The other name for lateral vestibular nucleus.

Déjèrine sign Acute pain in the neck on sneezing due to sudden increase in intraspinal pressure in cervical radiculopathy.

Déjèrine's anterior bulbar syndrome The other name for medial medullary nucleus, characterized by a crossed hemiplegic syndrome, hypoglossal nerve palsy on the ipsilateral side and pyramidal, lateral column, and posterior column signs in the contralateral side.

Déjèrine's cortical sensory syndrome Loss of proprioception, astereognosis, with preserved pain, temperature, and vibration sense in parietal lobe lesion.

Déjèrine's neurotabes A form of combined anterior and posterior radiculopathy where there is selective initial involvement of large fibres subserving deep sense associated with paraparesis in patients with syphilis.

Déjèrine's onion-peel sensory loss Sensory loss starting from mouth and nose and extending concentrically outward which is observed in lesions of the trigeminal nucleus, as happens in syringobulbia.

Déjèrine-Klumpke paralysis Lower brachial plexus palsy leading to weakness and wasting of muscles supplied by C8 and T1 usually following traction on the axilla. Horner's syndrome results from ablation of sympathetic fibers. This was a frequent complication of difficult breech delivery and traction on the following arm in earlier days. Incidentally, Klumpke was the wife of Dejerine and both were illustrious pupils of Jean Martin Charcot.

Déjèrine-Landouzy...	Déjèrine-Mouzon...
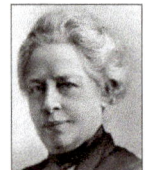	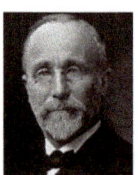
Augusta Dejerine Klumpke (1859–1927, France)	**Louis Théophile Joseph Landouzy (1845–1917, France)**
Déjèrine-Landouzy myopathy The other name for facioscapulohumeral dystrophy (Fig. D.3).	**Déjèrine-Mouzon syndrome** A parietal lobe syndrome with severe impairment of the primary modalities of sensation.

Figure D.3: Facioscapulohumeral dystrophy. Note prominent anterior axillary folds, winging of the scapulae and asymmetric involvement of the abdominal muscles, wasting being more pronounced in the left side

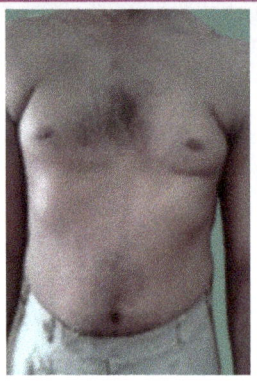
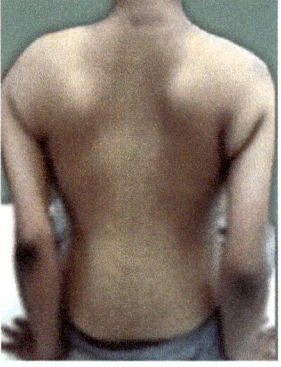

Déjèrine–Roussy syndrome

The other name of thalamic syndrome characterized by intense burning pain following thalamic stroke.

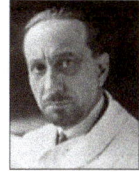

Gustave Roussy
(1874–1918, France)

Déjèrine–Sottas disease

Also known as progressive hypertrophic interstitial polyneuropathy of childhood, it is characterized by damage to the peripheral nerves resulting in muscle wasting. The onset is before 3 years of age with slow progression. The children have difficulty in walking and finally are wheel-chair bound. There is areflexia, sensory loss, muscular wasting, curved spine, deformities in foot and ataxia. There is mutation in MPZ, PMP22 and some other genes and is inherited as an autosomal dominant or recessive pattern. Biopsy shows hypertrophy of the interstitial connective tissue, giving rise to an *onion bulb appearance*. Nerve conduction studies show severe demyelinating neuropathy with gross reduction in conduction velocity with relative preservation of the amplitude.

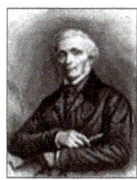

Jules Sottas (1866–1945, France)

Déjèrine-Thomas atrophy

The other name for olivopontocerebellar atrophy (Fig. D.4).

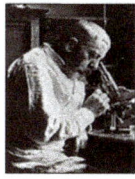

Joseph-Jules Dejerine
(1849–1917, France)

Figure D.4: MRI of spinocerebellar ataxia (SCA)

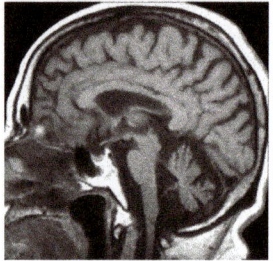

Denny-Brown syndrome Bronchogenic carcinoma associated with degeneration of dorsal root ganglion cells and primary degeneration of muscles. The other name for hereditary sensory and motor neuropathy type I.

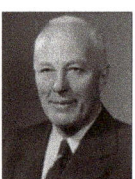

Derek Denny-Brown
(1901–1981, United States of America)

Denny-Brown-Foley's syndrome Benign fasciculation.

Descartes reflex The other name for menace reflex. This was the first reflex described in man.

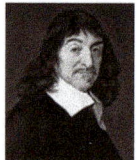

René Descartes
(1596–1650, France)

Descemet's membrane The posterior elastic lamina of the cornea, where copper is deposited in Wilson's disease resulting in the formation of the Kayser-Fleischer rings.

Devic's disease The combination of optic atrophy along with spastic paraparesis. Previously it was considered a variant of multiple sclerosis. Now it is treated as a definite entity and has been named *neuromyelitis optica*. The symptoms are loss of visual acuity, field defects or loss of color vision. The spinal cord pathology manifests as spastic paraparesis, severe paraesthesia, sensory loss, flexor spasms and sphincter incontinence. Causative factors include collagen vascular diseases, autoantibody syndromes, infections with varicella-zoster virus, Epstein–Barr virus and HIV infection, and exposure to antituberculous drugs. As opposed to multiple sclerosis, where cell mediated antibody produced by the T lymphocytes, humoral antibodies are targeted operators against myelin, known as NMO-IgG antibody in this condition. These antibodies attack the antigen, *aquaporin 4* in the astrocytes, which act as channels for the transport of water across the cell membrane. The astrocytes in proximity with the blood-brain barrier are rich in aquaporin 4 and the resultant damage leading to weakening of the barrier.

The criterion for diagnosis includes presence of opticneuritis and myelitis and supportive criteria suggests MRI of brain, not meeting the diagnosis of multiple sclerosis, involvement of more than 3 contiguous segments of spinal cord, and presence of anti-aquaporin 4 antibodies. Acute attacks are treated with intravenous methylprednisolone, corticosteroids or plasmapheresis. For prevention of attacks immunosuppression by azathioprine, mycophenolate mofetil, mitoxantrone, glatiramer acetate, and cyclophosphamide have been recommended. Rituximab, a monoclonal antibody has also been used with some success.

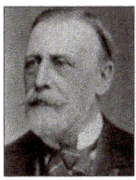

Eugène Devic
(1858–1930, France)

Dix-Hallpike maneuver A clinical test to determine whether the patient suffers from benign paroxysmal positional vertigo. The patient's head in supine position is suddenly extended at the edge of a table by the examiner and the test is considered positive if the subject complains of vertigo and there is appearance of nystagmus. A modification of the test is rotating the head of the patient by 45 degree to the side being tested. A negative result rules out positional nystagmus and hints at central lesion. This is also known as *Nylen-Barany test*.

Dorello's canal A bow-shaped microanatomical bony passage around the abducens nerve and the inferior petrosal sinus, as they enter the cavernous sinus. The upper wall of the canal is formed by the petrosphenoidal ligament. Sometimes, it is located at the tip of the petrous temporal bone.

Dostoyevsky epilepsy A rare variety of complex partial seizure, where the subject feels an ecstatic aura prior to an attack of seizure and, therefore, it has appropriately been termed, '*Ecstatic Epilepsy*'. It is said that Fyodor Dostoyevsky himself suffered from it, though others question whether this was a case of malingering.

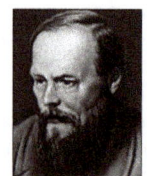

Fyodor Dostoyevsky (1821–1881, Russia)

Dravet syndrome Also known as severe myoclonic epilepsy of infancy, this variety of epilepsy is triggered by fever or hot temperature. Usually, there is febrile and afebrile seizures in the first year of life which later progresses to myoclonic epilepsy, partial seizures, ataxia, and psychomotor delay. Often there is autistic behavior, hyperactivity and impulsiveness. It is a cause of refractory seizure and often leads to severe status epilepticus. It is caused by nonsense mutations in SCN1A gene, which leads to impaired excitability of GABAergic neurons in the hippocampus. The genes are located in the long arm of chromosome 2 at 24.3 position. In the later stages the EEG shows slowing and generalized polyspikes. Stiripentol, a GABAergic agent has been found to be of some efficacy and ketogenic diet may also be tried. Cannabidiol is also of some value.

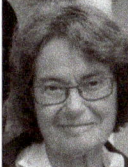

Charlotte Dravet (1936–till date, France)

Duane's syndrome A clinical condition where there is limitation of abduction of an eye and it is deviated medially in primary position by the unopposed action of the ipsilateral medial rectus. On attempted adduction of the affected eye, the globe retracts in to the socket along with narrowing of the palpebral fissure. The pathophysiology is controversial. Congenital absence of the abducens nucleus, congenital fibrosis of the lateral rectus muscle, or abnormal connection between the oculomotor and the abducent nerve are the possibilities.

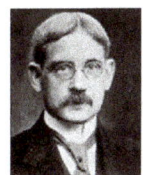

Alexander Duane (1858–1926, United States of America)

Duchenne sign Indrawing of the epigastrium with inspiration, a sign of diaphragmatic palsy.

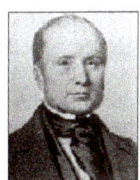

Guillaume-Benjamin-Amand Duchenne de Boulogne (1806–1875, France)

Duchenne's attitude Drooping of the shoulder with external rotation of the upper extremity due to paralysis of the trapezius muscle.

Duchenne's disease The other name for tabes dorsalis.

Duchenne's paralysis The other name for progressive bulbar palsy.

Duchenne-Aran palsy The other name for amyotrophic lateral sclerosis.

Duchenne-Griesinger disease This is more commonly known as Duchenne muscular dystrophy.

Dupré sign This refers to the fanning of the toes while eliciting the Babinski response. Thus it is a wrongly attributed credit to Babinski.

Dupuytren's canals The diploic spaces in the cranial bones.

Dürck's granuloma A granulomatous lesion found in the brain in malignant malaria. Petechial and ring hemorrhages are seen mostly in the white matte surrounding necrotic arterioles and venules. They tend to persist even after the blood cells are unaffected and are subsequently resolved by host response.

Duret hemorrhage Small punctate hemorrhagic spots in the brainstem in uncal herniation.

Durkan's compression test In carpal tunnel syndrome, the examiner places three fingers over the carpal tunnel which is kept in the supine position, and presses over it for 30 seconds. Appearance of pain and paraesthesia in the distribution of the median nerve in the wrist indicates positive test. Thus, the test is somewhat like Tinel's sign.

Dyke-Davidoff-Masson syndrome A congenital dysmorphic syndrome characterized by asymmetrical facial contour, thickening of calvarium due to hyperostosis frontalis interna, enlargement of frontal sinus, elevation of petrous bone ridge, hemiatrophy of cerebral hemisphere with unilateral dilatation of the lateral ventricle, and capillary malformations. It is clinically manifested as seizures (Fig. D.5).

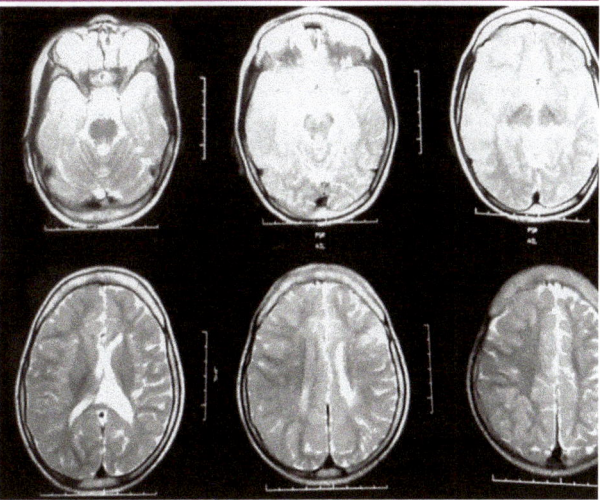

Figure D.5: Dyke-Davidoff-Masson syndrome: Note hyperostosis frontalis interna, atrophy of the left hemisphere, and dilatation of the lateral ventricle on the left side

SECTION E

Eagle syndrome Pain in the floor of the mouth caused by trauma induced by an unusually long styloid process of the temporal bone. It is usually seen in adults.

Eales disease A triad of retinitis proliferans, periphlebitis in the retina and angiopathia retinae juvenilis. There is recurrent vitreous and retinal hemorrhage in young patients. Sometimes myelopathy, seizures and focal neurological deficits are concomitant features.

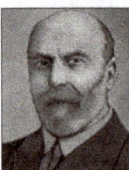

**Francis Henry Eales
(1852–1913, United Kingdom)**

Eastchester Clapping test

This is a test for hemineglect. In hemiparesis, if a person is asked to clap, he or she carries the unaffected hand to the opposite side and tap the hemiplegic hand. On the contrary, a subject with hemineglect, brings the hand to the midline and takes it back again to the original position.

Eaton–Lambert syndrome An autoimmune condition where weakness of muscles in the lower limbs is the predominant feature. This weakness tends to improve somewhat with exercise and exposure to high temperature worsens it. Autonomic symptoms like, dry mouth, constipation, postural hypotension, blurred vision and impaired sweating is seen in some cases. Power of the upper limb muscles improves on repeated forced gripping of hands, known as *Lambert's sign*. Antibodies are produced against voltage-gated calcium channels in the neuromuscular junctions. About 60% patients suffer from an underlying malignancy, most commonly, small cell carcinoma of lung, while other autoimmune diseases like, diabetes mellitus and hypothyroidism may be other associations. Sometimes it is associated with myasthenia gravis and HLA DR3-B8 gene in chromosome 6 may predispose to this condition. Usually a disease of the elderly, it is diagnosed by electromyography, where repetitive nerve stimulation at a high rate of 20 impulses per second for 10 seconds gives rise to classical incremental pattern, which may be even by 200% or more. This is attributed to the influx of calcium into the muscle cells. Single-fiber examination reveals increased jitter and blocking. Immunosuppressive therapy like intravenous immunoglobulin, prednisolone or azathioprine are of some use, as is plasmapheresis. 3,4-diaminopyridine and guanidine are also used occasionally.

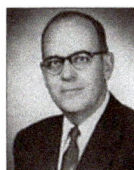

Lee Eaton (1905–1958, United States of America)

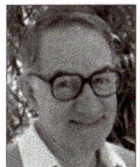

Edward Lambert (1915–2003, United States of America)

Eccles principle John Eccles of Australia trained in Oxford under Charles Scott Sherrington, used the stretch reflex as a model to study the functions of the synapse, already worked out by Sherrington. He used the simple principle that the synapse is constituted by a sensory neuron, the afferent arc from the muscle spindle and the efferent response from the motor neuron. A sensory impulse transmitted through the sensory nerve in the quadriceps femoris and a motor response evoked by the motor neuron innervating the muscle produces an excitatory postsynaptic potential (EPSP). On the contrary, if a similar current is passed through the antagonist muscle, the hamstrings, at the same time, an inhibitory postsynaptic potential (IPSP) is generated. The outcome of the movement of the muscle depends on the sum total of the two impulses. For this fundamental work, Eccles was awarded the Nobel Prize in 1963, along with Andrew Lloyd Hodgkin and Julius Huxley, who worked on the issue of sodium and potassium transfer across the cell membrane in order to produce a physiological response.

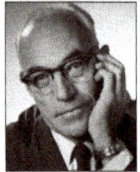

John Eccles
(1903–1997, Australia)

Edinger–Westphal nucleus

Also known as the accessory oculomotor nucleus, it is the parasympathetic preganglionic nucleus supplying the ciliary muscles and iris sphincter and helps in constricting the pupil, lens accommodation and convergence of the eyes. This paired nuclei constitute the posterior part of the oculomotor nucleus at the level of the superior colliculus. A curious function of the nucleus is that it responds to the emotional content of the face that a person sees and the pupils constrict or dilate accordingly. In recent times, it has been suggested that the nucleus does not contain cholinergic, preganglionic motor neurons, projecting into the ciliary ganglion. On the contrary, the neurons release peptides like, urocortin 1, with many central projections.

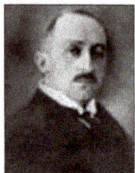

Ludwig Edinger
(1855–1918, Germany)

Egawa test A sign of ulnar nerve palsy, where the middle finger can be flexed but deviation radially or ulnarly is not possible. This happens due to paralysis of the interosseus muscle.

Egger syndrome
Joubert syndrome along with orofacio-digital congenital anomaly. Additional features are lobulated tongue, hamartomas in the mouth, and cyst in the posterior fossa. It is an autosomal recessive condition.

Ehlers-Danlos syndrome
Though not strictly a neurological malady, it should more appropriately be labelled as a disorder of connective tissue having a genetic basis. However, some neurological features are often observed in this condition like, carpal tunnel syndrome, Arnold-Chiari malformation, insensitivity to pain, quadriplegia from atlanto-axial dislocation due to laxity of ligaments, and dysautonomia. The laxity of the skin and hypermobility of the joints may masquerade as Marfan's syndrome.

Ekbom syndrome A delusional syndrome where the patients believe that their body is infested with parasites, maggots or insects. This is commonly found in schizophrenia and depression and females are affected more and it is often known as delusional parasitosis.

Ekbom-Wills syndrome The other name for restless leg syndrome. There is a strong urge to move the legs along with an unpleasant creeping sensation. This commonly occurs at night which awakens the patient from sleep and he wanders about which provides relief to some extent. Consequently, excessive daytime sleepiness, fatigue and depression are common accompaniments. Blood examination shows low iron, ferritin and transferrin. Pramipexole, levodopa, clonazepam and opioids are of some benefit.

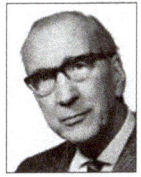

Karl-Axel Ekbom
(1907–1977, Sweden)

Elpenor syndrome A condition where a person after the ingestion of alcohol or narcotic drugs doze off to sleep and wake up in unfamiliar circumstances where they commit antisocial and destructive activities but remain amnestic and have little recollection of the events.

Elsberg phenomenon Compressive lesions near the foramen magnum may produce weakness of the ipsilateral shoulder and arm followed by weakness of the ipsilateral leg, then the contralateral leg, and finally the contralateral arm, a pattern that may begin in any of the four limbs.

Elsberg syndrome Polyradiculitis of the cauda equina with urinary retention and cerebrospinal fluid pleocytosis. It is usually a variant of acute inflammatory demyelinating polyradiculoneuropathy.

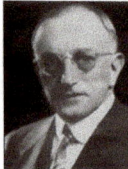

Charles Elsberg (1871–1948, United States of America)

Emery–Dreifuss syndrome A variety of X-linked muscular dystrophy where there is onset in childhood with muscular weakness, typically in the triceps and biceps and later involving the shoulder and the pelvic girdles. There is weakness of the facial muscles and rigidity of the paraspinal muscles. Cardiomyopathy and conduction block is common. There is early muscle contracture at the elbow, and neck without muscle pseudohypertrophy. The genetic locus is at Xq28.

Epley maneuver A maneuver to diagnose benign positional vertigo. This test leads to the displacement of the free floating otoliths from the posterior or anterior semicircular canals to the utricle and therefore, the cupola is no longer stimulated. The patient is relieved of vertigo.

Epworth sleepiness scale A questionnaire where a person rates subjectively the probability of falling asleep on a scale of increasing probability from 0 to 3 in 8 different situations and the value is added up. Values from 0 to 9 are considered normal, while values from 10 to 24 indicate serious sleep problem.

Erb myotonic reaction The prolonged contraction of a muscle resulting from faradic stimulation, when applied at the motor point.

Erb sign The phenomenon of hyperexitablity of nerves in tetany.

Erb's point The point behind the insertion of sternocleidomastoid muscle into the clavicle, used for the study of somatosensory evoked potential. The value obtained is designated as N9.

Erb's reaction of degeneration Persisting sensitivity of a muscle to galvanic stimulation but not to faradic stimulation following denervation.

Erb's reflex The other name for biceps reflex.

Erb's spastic paraparesis Syphilitic myelopathy involving the cervical cord due to pachymeningitis. It is sometimes referred as *Erb-Charcot syndrome*.

Erb's test Persisting sensitivity of muscles to galvanic but not faradic stimulation following denervation.

Erb–Duchenne paralysis Commonly known as Erb's palsy, it is caused by an injury to the upper trunk of the brachial plexus, particularly the C5 and C6 roots. Traction on the shoulder at the time of delivery like, shoulder dystocia, traction on the head, or pulling in breech presentation is a common cause. The nerves commonly involved are the suprascapular, musculocutaneous, and axillary nerves leading to lower motor neuron damage signs in the upper limb like, sensory loss, hypotonia, hyporeflexia, weakness and wasting. The affected arm hangs loosely by the side of the body in a medially rotated position, while the forearm is extended and pronated. This posture is known as *Waiter's Tip hand*.

Erb-Westphal sign The other name for absence of knee jerk in tabes dorsalis. Both of them described the sign in the January issue of *Deutsche Zeitschrift für Nervenheilkunde* in 1875. Erb's paper was published and Westphal wrote the editorial.

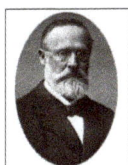

Wilhelm Heinrich Erb (1840–1921, Germany)

Ernest syndrome Characterized by facial pain due to inflammation of the tendon of the temporalis muscle, exacerbated by digital pressure over the stylomastoid ligament and relieved by injection of local anesthetic agent.

Escherich sign Periorbital and perioral muscular contraction in tetany induced by tapping the lips or tongue.

Espildora-Luque phenomenon Unilateral blindness with contralateral hemiplegia following embolism in ophthalmic artery, which leads to spasm in the middle cerebral artery on the same side.

Evans index A radiological sign about the ratio of the transverse diameter of the anterior horns of the lateral ventricles and the greatest internal diameter of the inner table of the skull in pneumoencephalography. This is decreased in hydrocephalus.

Ewald's law It states that the horizontal semicircular canal in the inner ear is maximally stimulated by movement of endolymph away from the ampulla and maximal stimulation of a semicircular canal results in the fast component of nystagmus toward the side of which it is stimulated.

Ewart phenomenon Elevation of the ptotic eyelid on swallowing, a synkinetic phenomenon following aberrant connection between the fibers of the facial and oculomotor nerves, the latter sending fibers to the levator palpebrae superioris muscle.

Exner's writing center A presumed cortical center concerned with writing located in the dominant frontal lobe in the middle frontal gyrus. It lies close to the frontal eye field anterior to the fibres supplying the hand in the primary motor cortex.

SECTION F

Fabry's disease A rare X-linked genetic disease of lysosomal storage, it is a variety of sphingolipidosis, where there is deficiency of the enzyme alpha galactosidase A due to mutation leading to to accumulation of a glycolipid, known as globotriosylceramide. Peripheral neuropathy, characterized by pain, tingling in the extremities, increased risk of childhood stroke, tinnitus, vertigo, and fatigue are common neurological symptoms and other organ systems like skin, heart, and kidneys are also affected. Angiokeratoma in the skin is characteristic. The diagnosis is confirmed by the assay of leukocyte alpha-galactosidase assay.

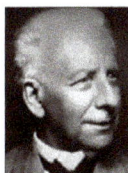

Johannes Fabry (1860–1930, Germany)

Fahn's pull test A classic test to observe the degree of postural instability in Parkinson's disease, where the patient stands with his back to the examiner. The examiner pulls at the shoulders suddenly and observes the number of steps the patient has to take in order to restore his stability. Care must be taken that he doesn't fall on the examiner and hurt. This was devised by Stanley Fahn from Columbia.

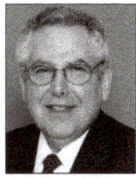

Stanley Fahn (1930–till date, United States of America)

Fahr disease Idiopathic basal ganglia calcification, which is inherited as a dominant condition characterized by deposits of calcium in basal ganglia. The genetic locus is identified at 14q position. Cerebral cortex may

Figure F.1: Fahr disease

also be involved. There may be seizures, involuntary movements and dementia. Bisphosphonates have been tried with some success in some patients (Fig. F.1).

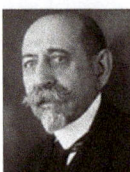

Karl Theodor Fahr (1877–1945, Germany)

Fazekas scale A radiological scoring system to quantify the amount of white matter T2 hyperintense lesions and severity due to small vessel ischemic disease. It divides the white matter into the periventricular and deep zones and is graded depending upon the size of the lesions. In periventricular white matter, 0 is credited if there is no lesion, 1 for pencil-thin lining, 2 for smooth halo and 3 for irregular signal extending into the deep white matter. The deep white matter lesions are graded as 0, if it is absent, 1 for punctate foci, 2 for the beginning of confluent lesions, and 3 for established conglomerated lesions.

Fazio-Londe syndrome A very rare inherited or familial variety of motor neuron disease where the muscles supplied by the lower cranial nerves are affected.

Dysphagia and dysarthria are common symptoms. It is linked to a genetic mutation in the SLC52A3 gene on chromosome 20p13.

Fergusson-Critchley syndrome Combination of spinocerebellar ataxia, spastic paraparesis, optic atrophy, supranuclear ophthalmoplegia, myoclonus and dementia. It is classified as an example of atypical motor neuron disease.

Finkel variety of spinal muscular atrophy A variety of spinal muscular atrophy in adult life, developing usually in the early 30s. There is mild to moderate proximal muscle weakness, tremor, cramps, twitching of the muscles and protuberant abdomen. In some subjects the sphincters are affected along with difficulty in deglutition. There is mutation in the VAPB gene and it is inherited as an autosomal dominant trait.

Fisher scale A scale for classifying subarachnoid hemorrhage by looking at the CT scan. In grade 1, no bleed is seen and incidence of symptomatic vasospasm is 21%. In grade 2, there is diffuse thin bleed of less than 1 mm, no clot and vasospasm is found in 25%. In grade 3, there is either layer of blood of more than 1 mm thickness or there is localized clot and the risk of vasospasm is 37%, while in grade 4, there is additional intracerebral or intraventricular bleed and vasospasm is found in 31% of cases.

Fischer's sign Paucity of facial emotional expression, which occurs in non-dominant hemispheric lesions, often accompanied by dysprosody.

Flatau's law The greater the length of the fibers in the spinal cord, the more peripheral they are placed. This is valid for the pyramidal and spinothalamic tracts but not for the fibers of the posterior column.

Flechsig's tract The other name for dorsal spinocerebellar tract.

Foix syndrome This is also known as *Marie-Foix-Alajouanine syndrome* or lateral pontine syndrome. It follows a brain stem vaso-occlusive disease in the perforating branches of basilar and anterior inferior cerebellar arteries. The clinical picture comprises in contralateral hemiparesis and hemianesthesia, ipsilateral limb ataxia, facial palsy and hearing loss.

Foix-Jefferson syndrome The other name for superior orbital fissure syndrome, where there is lesion in the 3rd, 4th, 5th and 6th cranial nerves in various combination, exophthalmos, and eyelid edema due to a tumor, aneurysm, or thrombosis of the cavernous sinus.

Forel's decussation The ventral tegmental decussation between the red nuclei.

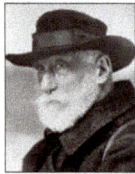

**Auguste-Henri Forel
(1848–1931, Switzerland)**

Foster–Kennedy syndrome One of the most classical and unmistakable syndrome complexes in neurology. It is usually seen in olfactory groove meningioma, which compresses the ipsilateral optic nerve, and the olfactory nerve roots emerging from the cribriform plate of ethmoid bone. Resultantly, the unilateral anosmia and optic atrophy and the raised intracranial pressure caused in the process, obstructs the flow of cerebrospinal fluid which leads to papilloedema in the contralateral eye. This is the first ever syndrome described with the help of the ophthalmoscope. The presence of such ocular findings in the absence of any space-occupying lesion is known as *Pseudo Foster Kennedy syndrome* and most commonly results from non-arteritic ischemic optic neuropathy.

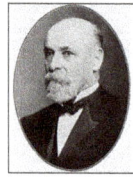

**Robert Foster Kennedy
(1884–1952, United Kingdom)**

Fothergill syndrome The other name for trigeminal neuralgia.

Foville's syndrome A brain stem vascular syndrome characterized by occlusive lesions in the perforating branches of the basilar artery in the pons. This is characterized by facial palsy and

Foville-Wilson syndrome A term used to describe the impairment of lateral convergence often found in disseminated sclerosis.

Frankel scale A scale devised for patients with spinal injury.

Fregoli syndrome It is a condition, closely related to Capgras' syndrome, where a familiar person is felt as a stranger, in spite of close resemblance to the person in question. This often occurs in advanced schizophrenia.

Frenzel's glasses A diagnostic tool used to evaluate nystagmus. The pair of glasses are biconvex of more than +20 diopters, like a magnifying glass which blurs visual fixation and thus, nystagmus is rendered evident.

Frey's syndrome Also known as Dupuy's syndrome, this is a condition where there is gustatory sweating in neck, cheek, jaw and adjacent areas. This occurs following synkinesis between autonomic fibers in the glossopharyngeal and vagus nerve, particularly in neck trauma and subsequent dissection.

Fricht Lundborg disease A common cause of progressive myoclonic epilepsy. It commonly affects children between the ages of 6 to 16 years and is characterized by tonic clonic and myoclonic seizures. It is an autosomal recessive disorder with mutation in the cystatin B gene but recent studies have shown that an increased number of dopamine receptors are found the brain in this condition and this might explain the occurrence of higher incidence of myoclonic jerks. It is also postulated that the lack of cystatin B leads to a decrease in the inhibitory GABAergic neurons in this disease, rendering the cells in the hippocampus excitable, which explains the incidence of various kinds of seizures. Since cystatin B is a neuroprotective agent, its absence exposes the neuronal vulnerability to damage after the seizures.

Friedreich ataxia The condition was first brought to light by Nikolaus Friedreich of Germany in 1863 and is the first form of hereditary ataxia described in the world. (The reader is referred to any standard textbook of neurology)

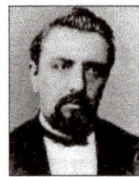

**Nikolaus Friedreich
(1825–1882, Germany)**

Froin's syndrome A triad of xanthochromia, high protein in cerebrospinal fluid and hypercoagulability of the fluid in tumor of the spinal cord. Stasis of cerebrospinal fluid in the subarachnoid space leads to exudation from the tumor and activation of coagulation factors. Spinal neurofibroma is a common cause. *Pseudo-Froin's syndrome* refers to stagnation of the fluid distal to spinal block due to disc prolapse.

Froment's sign In suspected ulnar nerve palsy, the patient is asked to hold a piece of paper in between his thumb and the index finger in pinch grip. The examiner then attempts to pull it away. In ulnar nerve palsy due to paralysis of adductor pollicis, supplied by the nerve, the paper shall slip out easily and in order to compensate, the patient will bring his flexor pollicis longus and interossei into operation. Resultantly, the thumb will be seen in flexed position. If the metatarsophalangeal joint is hyperextended, it is known as *Jeanne's sign*.

Fuchs' phenomenon A phenomenon of regenerative synkinesis where there is paradoxical lid retraction associated with ocular movement during recovery from damage to oculomotor nerve. This is also known as *pseudo-Graefe phenomenon*.

Fukuda stepping test A test for assessment of unilateral vestibular lesion presenting as dizziness. A wide circle is drawn on the floor and the patient is blindfolded. He is then asked to take a few steps forward in a straight line the arms being outstretched. In unilateral vestibular lesion the subject will sway to the side of the lesion.

Fukuyama muscular dystrophy A variety of congenital

muscular dystrophy described originally from Japan, where the brain, muscles and the eyes are affected. It is an autosomal recessive disorder with muscular dystrophy, cognitive impairment, contractures, and ptosis. The mutation is in the FTKN gene which codes for the protein, fukutin.

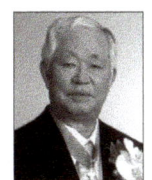

Yukio Fukuyama (1928–2014, Japan)

SECTION G

Galen's vein Also known as the great cerebral vein, it is a short vein formed by the union of the two internal cerebral veins and basal veins of Rosenthal. It is in the quadrigeminal cistern and curves backward and upward along the posterior border of the splenium of the corpus callosum and drains into the confluence of the inferior sagittal sinus and the straight sinus. It receives tributaries from the callosal veins, precentral cerebellar vein, superior cerebellar veins and the inferior cerebral veins.

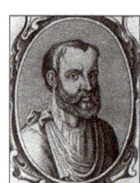

Claudius Galenus, often known as Galen of Pergamon (129–216AD, Greece)

Galvanic current A variety of current which occurs in the presence of two or more dissimilar metals in an electrolyte or saltwater environment and can be measured. It is also defined as the unidirectional current of an electric charge. This was first brought to light by Luigi Aloisio Galvani, an Italian physicist and physician in 1780.

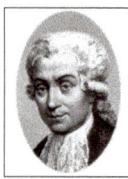

Luigi Galvani (1737–1798, Italy)

Ganser syndrome Often known as nonsense syndrome, the patient provides approximate answer to a question, which is close but not appropriate. This occurs in severe depression, schizophrenia, head injury, or in malingering. Since the answers are always in response to the examiner's questions and never spontaneous, and since they are somewhat meaningful, it suggests that the patient has grasped the meaning. Sometimes it is seen among prisoners who presumably use this strategy for benefit and therefore, it is also known as *prison psychosis*. It is a thought to be a reaction to extreme stress and is a variety of dissociative disorder.

Garcin syndrome Paralysis of almost all the cranial nerves of one side without any evidence of long tract signs. This is commonly found in malignant infiltration from sarcoma of the nasopharynx.

Gardner syndrome The other name for type 2 neurofibroma, a dominantly inherited bilateral vestibular schwannoma without any peripheral stigmata. The chromosome 22 is implicated and the function of the tumor suppressor factor Merlin is abnormal, leading to cell growth.

Gardner's hypothesis A hypothesis to explain the pathophysiology of syringomyelia in 1958. He proposed that an obstruction to the flow of cerebrospinal fluid outflow from the 4th ventricle diverts the fluid pulse wave into the central canal. This was thus named *'water hammer theory'*. This leads to creation of longitudinal fluid-filled cavities inside the spinal cord. This hydrodynamic theory held much water for about 20 years. It has recently been questioned, though magnetic resonance imaging studies lend credence to many aspects of Gardner's view.

Garland's syndrome The other name for diabetic amyotrophy described by Hugh Garland from Leeds, in 1951. The first case he described presented with extensor plantar response and Garland felt that the lesion was in the spinal cord, and hence he called the condition, diabetic myelopathy. However, in later series, he found the plantar response consistently flexor and he coined the term diabetic amyotrophy, which is asymmetrical, painful, proximal neuropathy in the thighs. Classically, the knee jerk is lost earlier than the ankle jerk in this variety of diabetic neuropathy.

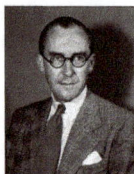

Hugh Garland (1903–1967, United Kingdom)

Gastaut syndrome A variety of epilepsy where there is unilateral convulsion, hemiparesis and epigastric or pharyngeal aura in children. However, Gastaut is more famous for his association with William Gordon Lennox in describing *Lennox-Gastaut syndrome*.

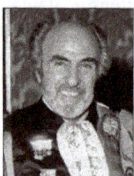

Henri Jean Pascal Gastaut (1915–1995, France)

Gaucher cells Swollen cells with cerebrosides along with a foamy appearance. Incidentally, Gaucher was a dermatologist from France.

Gaucher's disease A disorder of metabolism where there is accumulation of cerebrosides in various organs in the body. Clinically, it is characterized by hepatosplenomegaly, seizures, myoclonus and dementia. It is an autosomal recessive disease and the chromosome implicated is 1q22, while the mutation is in the GBA gene. There are three varieties and in type 1, the nervous system is not affected. Type 2 is prognostically the worst variety.

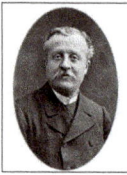

Philippe Charles Ernest Gaucher (1854–1918, France)

Gennari's lines This is a band of myelinated axons running parallel to the surface of the cerebral cortex in the calcarine sulcus of the occipital lobe. They represent the axons derived from the thalamus to the layer IV of the visual cortex. Gennari described these bands at a time while he was a student in Padua. They represent the outer portion of the *bands of Baillarger*.

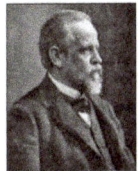

Francesco Gennari
(1750–1797, Italy)

Gerhardt's law In paralysis of the vocal cord due to lesion in the recurrent laryngeal nerve, it assumes mid-position between complete abduction and adduction.

Gerhardt's syndrome Bilateral adductor paralysis of the vocal cord due to lesion at the base of the skull. The condition is also referred to the identical pathology in multiple system atrophy.

Gerstmann's syndrome Constellation of right-left disorientation, acalculia, finger agnosia and agraphia due to a lesion in the dominant angular and supramarginal gyrus in the parietal lobe.

Gerstmann-Schilder syndrome Apraxia of gait and disequilibrium following lesion in the frontal lobe. The condition resembles cerebellar ataxia. It is somewhat similar to *Bruns' apraxia* and possibly results from damage to the frontopontocerebellar fibers.

Gerstmann–Straussler–Scheinker disease A rare, familial and fatal neurodegenerative disorder which resembles transmissible spongiform encephalopathy and is considered a Prion disease. Clinically, it presents like spinocerebellar ataxia with parkinsonian features, pyramidal signs, rapidly progressive dementia and impaired smooth pursuit movement of the eyes. It is an autosomal dominant disorder and the mutation is at chromosome 20.

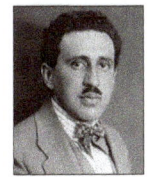

Josef Gerstmann
(1887–1969, Austria)

Geschwind–Galaburda hypothesis Sex differences in cognitive abilities is related to lateralization of brain function. Maturation in the cerebral hemispheres is mediated by circulating testosterone levels and sexual maturation acts to fix the hemispheres at different relative stages of development after puberty. According to this theory, male brains mature later than females, and the left hemisphere matures later than the right.

Geschwind-Gastaut phenomenon A feature of complex partial seizure characterized by hypergraphia, hyperreligiosity, hypersexuality and hyperviscosity or circumstantiality.

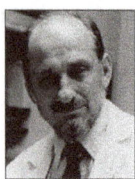

Norman Geschwind (1926–1984, United States of America)

Gibbs' hypsarrhythmia A peculiar kind of epileptiform discharges, also known as mountainous arrhythmia with infantile spasms and developmental delay. The spasm consists of *salaam attack*, coined by Charles Bell of United Kingdom, where the neck, upper torso, and the upper limbs flex suddenly. All of these features constitute the core features of *West's syndrome*. It should be of some historical interest to note that Charles West, a physician, found these unusual features in his son, and consulted Sir Charles Bell. He sent a letter to *The Lancet*, describing his son's malady, which was published in 1841. Hypsarrhythmia is diagnosed with the patient in the awake state.

Godfredsen syndrome A rare condition where there is abducent nerve palsy along with ipsilateral hypoglossal nerve palsy. Usually it is due to invasion from a mass at the clivus, extending to the cavernous sinus and the retropharyngeal space, which in turn, leads to the involvement of the two disparate cranial nerves which are not in close proximity in their intracerebral course.

Golgi apparatus This organelle collects and dispatches protein products received from the endoplasmic reticulum. Proteins synthesized their are packed in small vesicles which fuse with the Golgi apparatus. It is also concerned with lipid transport and lysosome formation.

Golgi corpuscles Cutaneous end organs for touch sensation.

Golgi stain A stain technique for visualizing nerve tissue under light microscope. It was discovered by Camillo Golgi, an Italian neuroscientist and a Nobel Laureate in 1906, along with Ramón y Cajal.

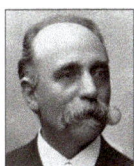
Camillo Golgi
(1844–1926, Italy)

Goll's tract The other name for fasciculus gracilis, carrying proprioceptive fibers from the lower limb and the lower half of the trunk in the posterior column, lying medial to the tract of Burdach, or fasciculus cuneatus.

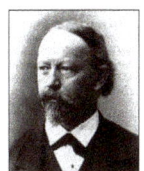
Friedrich Goll
(1829–1903, Switzerland)

Gömöri's trichrome stain A stain used to diagnose histologically mitochondrial myopathies by the demonstration of ragged red fibers.

Gonda's sign Also known as Allen's sign, this is seen in lesions of the pyramidal tract damage where dorsiflexion of the great toe is seen in response to downward stretching and sudden release of the second toe.

Gordon's reflex Demonstration of the upgoing toe in corticospinal tract disorder where the reflex is elicited by squeezing the Achilles tendon.

Gottron's sign Also known as Gottron's papule, it is a scaly, patchy redness over the knuckles seen in patients with dermatomyositis, an inflammatory muscle disorder, and considered a pathognomonic sign. Skin biopsy shows acanthosis, hyperkeratosis with focal vacuolar alteration of the basal-cell layer, and perivascular inflammatory infiltrates.

Gower's sign A clinical sign to detect weakness of the proximal muscles in the lower limbs. The patient while getting up from the floor, puts his hands on the floor, then on the legs, thighs and gets up. It is often known as '*climbing on one's knees*'. This is found classically in Duchenne muscular dystrophy but it can be positive in any condition where the proximal muscles of the lower limbs are weak, as in rickets and osteomalacia.

Gower's tetanoid chorea The older name for Wilson's disease

Gower's tract The other name for anterior spinothalamic tract.

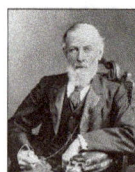

William Richard Gowers (1845–1915, United Kingdom)

Gower–Laing myopathy A variety of distal myopathy in childhood where there is weakness in the anterior compartment of the leg. The subject cannot lift the big toe and contracture of the Achilles tendon leads to toe walking and high stepping gait. Later weakness appears in the upper limbs and sometime, in the neck and face. It is inherited as an autosomal dominant disorder and the mutation in the MYH7 gene.

Gradenigo's syndrome Combination of abducens nerve palsy along with anesthesia in the distribution of the ophthalmic branch of the trigeminal nerve due to a lesion in the petrous part of the temporal bone, usually from osteitis. The abducent nerve hooks around the apex of the petrous bone and the trigeminal ganglion is lodged in a small fossa in the anterior surface of the petrous bone.

Graefe's sign The lag in the decent of the upper eyelid in thyrotoxicosis and myotonic conditions. The *pseudo-Graefe's sign* refers to the elevation of the upper eyelid on looking down as a result of aberrant nerve regeneration following trauma to the oculomotor nerve.

Greenfield's disease The other name for infantile metachromatic leukodystrophy.

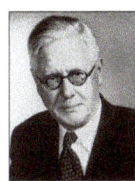

Godwin Greenfield
(1884–1958, United Kingdom)

Gudden's atrophy Secondary degeneration of the thalamic nuclei following destruction of certain cortical areas.

Gudden's commissure The tract that connects the inferior quadrigeminal body and the medical geniculate bodies of the two sides.

Gudden's inferior commissure Fibres of optic tract.

Gudden's law The degeneration of the proximal end of a divided peripheral nerve proceeds centripetally.

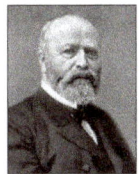

Johann Bernhard Aloys von Gudden (1824–1886, Germany)

Gudden's tract Other name for the transverse peduncular tract.

Gudden-Wanner sign Shortening of the bone conduction time of a tuning fork over bony cranial scars.

Guillain–Mollaret triangle An imaginary triangle created by the red nucleus, inferior olivary nucleus and the contralateral dentate nucleus. A lesion in this triangle leads to the development of palatal tremor. Incidentally, the olivary nucleus is hypertrophied in this condition and thus it is an example of an organ undergoing hypertrophy in a degenerative condition.

Guyon's canal syndrome As the ulnar nerve crosses the wrist, it enters the tunnel formed by the pisiform and the hamate bone and the ligament which connects these bones. The nerve can be trapped in this canal and tingling and paraesthesia in the medial one and a half fingers is the presentation.

SECTION H

Hachinski ischemic score A 13-item clinical scoring system to differentiate degenerative from vascular dementia. The points to consider are abrupt onset, emotional incontinence, stepwise deterioration, prior history of hypertension, fluctuating coarse, history of strokes, nocturnal confusion, evidence of atherosclerosis, relative preservation of personality, focal neurological symptoms, depression, focal neurological sigs, and somatic complaints. Some of the items are assigned values of 1, while others are labeled as 2. A score above 7 suggests vascular dementia, while in Alzheimer's disease, the score is below 3.

Hachinski's sign A subtle sign in minor strokes and transient ischemic attacks where the thumb goes up on scratching the palm. It is somewhat like the Babinski sign in the lower limbs and is considered a reliable sign in various studies.

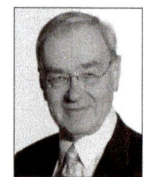

**Vladimir Hachinski
(1941–till date, Canada)**

Haenel sign Absence of pain when the closed eyes are pressed firmly by the fingers. It is a sign of neurosyphilis. Utmost caution is necessary since it may produce hypotension and bradykinesia due to vagal stimulation.

Hakim–Adam syndrome The other name for normal pressure hydrocephalus. The condition was the doctoral thesis of Salómon Hakim under the supervision of Raymond Delacy Adams and it was brought to light in 1965.

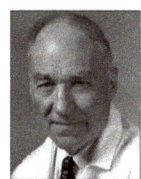

Raymond Delacy Adams (1911–2008, United States of America)

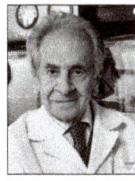

Salomón Hakim (1922–2011, United States of America

Hallervorden–Spatz disease

Recently named pantothenate kinase-associated neurodegeneration or neurodegeneration with brain iron accumulation 1, it is a neurodegenerative condition with features of parkinsonism, dystonia, tremor, spasticity, seizures, toe walking, and dementia. The onset is in childhood and progresses till adulthood leading to early death. It is an autosomal recessive disorder caused by a mutant gene, PANK2 located at chromosome 20p 13-p12.3. The genetic defect leads to the deposition of iron in the basal ganglia, leading to what is often known as '*Eye of the Tiger sign*', where in the globus pallidus there is a symmetrical central high intensity signal in the T2-weighted image. In India it is commonly seen in the Agarwal community. Iron chelating therapy with agents like desferrioxamine has not been successfully and therefore, the recent trend is to treat the patients with pantothenate.

Julius Hallervorden and Hugo Spatz of Germany described the condition first at the time of the 2nd World War and therefore, the eponym was rightfully conferred on them. However, both of them were staunch supporters of Hitler's Nazi party and they supervised the death of many Jew children in order to collect their brain for their study. It is even on record that Hallervorden once said, '*It doesn't matter where the brain comes from, as long as they come... the more the better*'. This abominable act on the part of these two gifted pathologists was highly criticized and they were calumniated to the extent that the eponym has finally been expunged from the medical literature and replaced by a lucid term '*pantothenate kinase-associated neurodegeneration*', in order to indicate the etiopathogenesis.

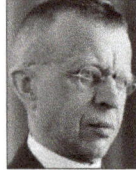

**Julius Hallervorden
(1882–1965, Germany)**

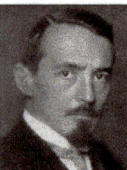

**Hugo Spatz
(1888–1969, Germany)**

Halliday's pattern reversal test A method to study visual evoked potential status, where the checker board pattern, akin to chess board in the television changes, black changing to white, and then white to black periodically, while the patient looks at the screen. An electrode is placed in the scalp and the tracing recorded on the screen. This test is great diagnostic value in demyelinating illnesses, and axonopathy in the anterior visual pathway. Half screen test can also be done to know the status of the optic tracts.

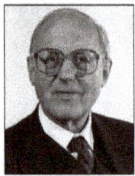

**Anthony Martin Halliday
(1926–2008, United Kingdom)**

Hammond's disease The other name for athetosis, it manifests months after birth, particularly with prematurity, along with slow, writhing, purposeless movements mainly affecting the hands and face, with forced laughter and crying. The joints are stretchable and spasticity develops soon. Both autosomal dominant and recessive forms have been described. Intelligence is normal. Lesions of the midbrain, thalamic nuclei, pallidostratium, and internal capsule are the cause of this disorder. Premature infants are frequently affected.

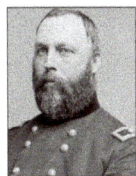

William Alexander Hammond (1828–1900, United States of America)

Hanes sign If a normal subject is asked to whistle, usually he smiles immediately after the act. This is classically absent in Parkinson's disease, presumably owing to hypomimia.

Harding's classification of cerebellar ataxia A classification of autosomal dominant cerebellar ataxias or ADCAs, based on clinical features. These are a clinically and genetically heterogeneous group of disorders characterized by a slowly progressive cerebellar syndrome presenting as ataxia of gait, dysarthria, peripheral neuropathy, and oculomotor disorders due to primary cerebellar degeneration. The degenerative process can be limited to the cerebellum or can involve the retina, optic nerve, pons, medulla, basal ganglia, cerebral cortex, spinal tracts, or peripheral nerves. If the optic nerve, pons and medulla, basal ganglia, cortex, spinal cord, and peripheral nerves are involved apart from the cerebellum, it is designated as ADCA type I, if the retina is involved, ADCA type II, and if it is pure cerebellar degeneration, it is called ADCA III. Incidentally, it must be borne in mind that the other commonly used term spinocerebellar ataxias, or SCAs is an entity, reserved for the genetics of these disparate condition, like SCA1 in chromosome 6, SCA2 in chromosome 12, SCA3 in chromosome 14, and so on and so forth, while ADCA is purely a clinical description. The general view held is that SCA2 is the commonest variety in India, which was first reported by Wadia et al, from Mumbai. However, there are ethnic variations in the country.

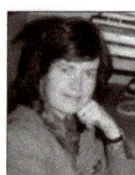

Anita Elizabeth Harding
(1952–1995, United Kingdom)

Harris' sign The other name for internuclear ophthalmoplegia. Wilfred Harris became the first President of Association of British Neurologists, with Gordon Holmes as the Secretary, and Kinnier Wilson as the treasurer in 1932.

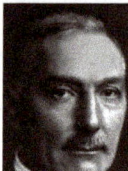

Wilfred Harris
(1869–1960, United States of America)

Hashimoto's encephalitis Also known as steroid responsive encephalopathy associated with autoimmune thyroiditis, this is characterized by encephalopathy and thyroid autoimmune disorder. Other features include, personality changes, delusion, aggression, disorientation, myoclonic jerks, psychosis, seizures, sleep problems, etc. Auto-antibodies of alpha-enolase has been found to be associated with this condition and increased thyroid-stimulating hormone is an important finding. Thyroid antibodies like anti thyroid peroxidase antibodies like anti-TPO, anti thyroid microsomal antibodies and antithyroglobulin antibodies are also elevated. Most of the patients respond to steroids or immunosuppressant therapy.

Hawkin's test An impingement test where pain is reproduced by trapping of the rotator cuff tendons between the head of the humerus and the acromion process. The arm is abducted, externally rotated, and internally rotated forcefully. Pain is felt in fibromyalgia and related conditions.

Head zones These are bands of cutaneous hyperesthesia associated with acute or chronic inflammation of the viscera, described by Henry Head of London.

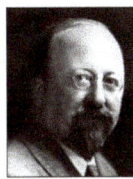

Henry Head
(1861–1940, United Kingdom)

Head's negative after reaction The inspiratory effort made even after respiration stops following inflation of the lungs of an experimental animal (*Head's Paradoxical Reflex*).

Head's zones Zones of hyperalgesia of skin, associated with visceral disease, for instance, pain in the tip of the right shoulder in diseases of the gallbladder.

Head-Riddoch syndrome A syndrome occurring in quadriplegic patients consisting of bradycardia, hypertension, pupillary dilatation, sweating, nasal stuffiness, blurred vision, and headache.

Heidenhain syndrome This is a variant of Creutzfeldt–Jakob disease, where visual manifestations dominate the clinical picture persists throughout the disease course. These include disturbed perception of colors or structures, optical hallucinations, cortical blindness and visual anosognosia. The most pronounced neuropathological changes are localized to the occipital lobe.

Heimann-Bielschowsky phenomenon A feature peculiar to dissociated vertical deviation.

Hering's law This law of equal innervation states that in conjugate saccadic eye movement the muscles responsible for the movement of each eye are supplied equally by the oculomotor nerves.

Heschl gyrus The transverse temporal lobe behind the insula on the medial and superior aspect of the superior temporal gyrus which is thought to be concerned with hearing.

Heubner's artery Recurrent artery arising from the proximal A2 or distal A1 segment, or at the level of the optic chiasma of the anterior cerebral artery.

Hilton's law The same trunks of nerves whose branches supply groups of muscles moving a joint, also send a twig to the skin overlying the joint.

Hirano bodies Intracellular aggregates of proteins seen in Alzheimer's disease and Creutzfeldt–Jakob disease. These were first described in the CA1 segment of the hippocampus in amyotrophic lateral sclerosis and parkinsonism-dementia complex of Guam. Some consider these as natural accompaniments of aging having no special clinical significance.

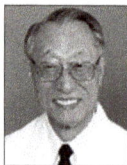

**Asao Hirano
(1926–till date, Japan)**

Hirayama disease A variety of unilateral focal motor neuron disease affecting young subjects. The onset is insidious with wasting of small muscles of the hand and the disease stabilizes after 2–5 years. Sensory features are remarkably absent and fasciculations are rare. Electromyography shows denervation. It is a type of chronic partial cervical myelopathy related to flexion movement of the neck and chronic ischemic changes in the area supplied by the anterior spinal artery induced by flexion injury causes necrosis of the anterior horn cells in the lower cervical cord. MRI of the cervical spine in extension and flexion is diagnostic and there is forward migration of the posterior wall of the dura mater. The posterior epidural space is enlarged in flexion and a high signal intensity crescentic space is seen. The space is narrowed in extension.

Such forms of focal amyotrophy have also been described from India. Gourie-Devi from Bangalore described a similar sort of condition, named *Monomelic Amyotrophy* (Fig. H.1) and follow-up studies conducted by her group emphasized the benign nature of the disease, its restriction to one limb, lack of involvement of cranial nerves, and pure lower motor involvement. She suggested the terms, brachial and crural monomelic amyotrophy, based on the involvement of the upper or lower limb, respectively. Prabhakar and Chopra from Chandigarh described wasting in one lower limb and called it *Wasted Leg Syndrome*.

Hirayama disease

Figure H.1: Hirayama disease. Note increase in posterior epidural space during flexion

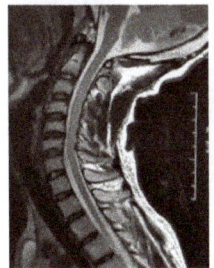
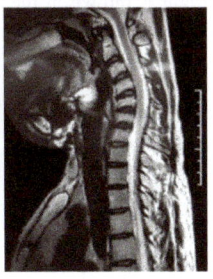

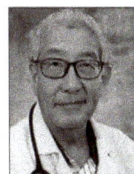

Keizo Hirayama
(1929–till date, Japan)

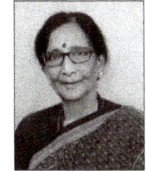

M Gourie-Devi
(1938–till date, India)

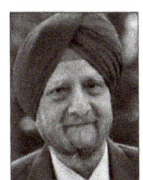

Jagjit Singh Chopra
(1935–2019, India)

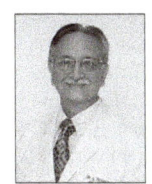

Sudesh Prabhakar
(1949–till date, India)

Hirschberg test A test to assess the presence of strabismus in a subject. Light is thrown in the eyes and the reflection from the cornea is observed. With normal ocular alignment, the light reflex is nasal from the center of cornea, since the cornea is a temporally tilted convex structure. The light reflex, emanating from the cornea is symmetrical in a normal person. In exotropia, where the eye is turned out, the light shines through the medial aspect of the cornea, while in esotropia, where it is turned inwards, the light reflex appears at the lateral aspect.

Hoehn and Yahr scale A scale devised by Melvin Yahr and Margaret Hoehn from Mount Senoi hospital in 1967, to assess degree of advancement and the resultant disability. It is rated from stage I to stage V in terms of the degree of severity. Stage I refers to mild unilateral involvement, while stage V is the non ambulatory, wheel-chair bound state.

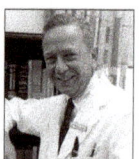

Melvin Yahr (1917–2004, United States of America)

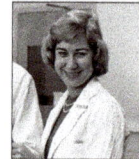

Margaret Hoehn (1931–2005, United States of America)

Hoffman syndrome Hypertrophy of the calf muscles in hypothyroidism in adults. In children, the same feature is known as *Kocher–Debré–Semelaigne syndrome*.

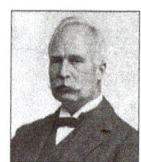

Johann Hoffman (1857–1919, Germany)

Hoffman's reflex A sign of pyramidal tract lesion where flicking the terminal phalanx of the middle finger, held in the flexed posture, leads to flexion and adduction of the terminal phalanx of the thumb. Sometimes it is erroneously referred to as the *Babinski reflex in the upper limb*. It is also known as *Hoffman's sign*.

There is one more Hoffman's reflex in the field of electrophysiology. The H reflex, derived from his name assesses the integrity of the spinal reflex at the level of L5 and S1 segment of the spinal cord. Its absence indicates breach in the reflex pathway and S1 radiculopathy It is often considered the electrophysiological equivalent of the ankle jerk.

Holmes rebound phenomenon A sign of cerebellar dysfunction where if the subject's outstretched upper limb is flexed at the elbow against resistance by the examiner and is released suddenly, the hand flings abnormally upwards and in severe cases the subject may even fall behind injuring himself. Care must be taken that the ataxic upper limb does not hit against the patient's face and one hand of the examiner is therefore, kept in front of the face in order to avoid the inadvertent injury.

Holmes' dermatome map The standard dermatomal distribution pattern, as shown in all books on neurology for testing the exteroceptive or spinothalamic sensation. This was devised in 1911. However, there are controversies regarding the primary designer of this map.

Holmes' syndrome A variety of inherited ataxia with degeneration of the olivary nucleus.

Holmes' tremor Coarse rubral tremor, described by Gordon Holmes in 1904. It is a misnomer since it is not caused by lesion in the red nucleus. The lesion is in the nigrostriatal pathway. It is also known as *Bat's Wing tremor*.

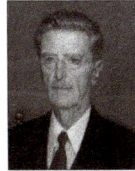

Gordon Morgan Holmes (1876–1965, United Kingdom)

Holmes–Adie syndrome A syndrome of tonically dilated pupil which reacts slowly to light with preserved accommodation. It starts in one eye and with time tends to be bilateral. The pupils become smaller with time. Classically, a dilute solution of pilocarpine which has no effect in the normal pupil, leads to pupillary constriction due to denervation supersensitive or *Cannon's law*. The knee or the ankle jerks are characteristically absent. It is caused by damage to the postganglionic parasympathetic fibers in the ciliary ganglion in the orbit following a viral infection. In some instances familial cases conforming to an autosomal dominant inheritance has been observed. John Adie, an Australian immigrant, was the Registrar to Gordon Holmes in Queen Square, London and he described the pupillary abnormalities, while the original case Holmes described had reduced knee jerk, though later workers showed that the ankle jerk is more commonly affected.

Holmes-Logan syndrome A hereditary dysmorphic syndrome, comprising in failure of growth, optic atrophy, ophthalmoplegia, areflexia, choreoathetosis and mental and motor retardation.

Hooper Visual Organization Test A test for constructional ability, which includes a series of line drawings of increasing complexity, that have been cut into a variety of separate segments. The subject has to identify the object by mentally organizing the various segments.

Hoover's sign A clinical sign to distinguish organic from hysterical hemiplegia. The examiner puts one palm below the heel of the paralyzed limb and asks the patient to lift the normal limb against resistance. In organic hemiplegia, the paralyzed limb goes up but in malingering the paralyzed heel presses upon the palm.

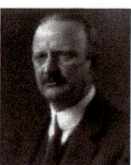

Charles Franklin Hoover (1865–1927, United States of America)

Hoppe-Goldflam disease The other name for myasthenia gravis.

Horner syndrome A constellation of signs like partial ptosis, meiosis, enophthalmos, anhidrosis, and loss of ciliospinal reflex. It is caused by sympathetic denervation following damage to the sympathetic trunk. In some cases, the conjunctiva and the face may appear bloodshot due to capillary dilatation. In congenital Horner's syndrome hair on the affected side may appear straight and the iris is heterochromic. It may be caused by central lesions, manifested by anhidrosis of face, body and limb and caused by syringomyelia, multiple sclerosis, Wallenberg's syndrome, etc, pre ganglionic lesion, characterized by anhidrosis of the face only due to cervical rib, thyroidectomy, carcinoma of thyroid, Pancoast's tumor, Klumpke's paralysis, thoracic outlet syndrome, etc, or post ganglionic lesion, where there is no anhidrosis. The common causes are migrainous headaches, cluster headache, carotid dissection, cavernous sinus thrombosis, sympathectomy for Buerger's disease, or middle ear infection. In children the common causes are birth trauma and neuroblastoma. The condition is diagnosed by the cocaine drop test. When 4% cocaine is instilled in the palpebral fissure, it blocks the reuptake of norepinephrine in the normal eye and there is dilatation of the pupil. In Horner's syndrome, lack of cocaine in the synaptic cleft leads to failure in mydriasis. The alpha-agonist apraclonidine is a more modern agent and leads to increased mydriasis due to denervation supersensitivity. However, in order to distinguish between central and peripheral lesion, Paredrine test is utilized. If the lesion is peripheral, it causes mydriasis; in central lesion, it has no effect upon the pupil.

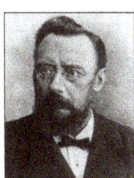

Johann Friedrich Horner (1831–1886, Switzerland)

Horsley's sign The finding that axillary temperature is higher on the side affected in hemiplegia.

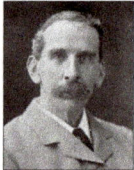

Victor Alexander Horsley (1857–1916, United Kingdom)

Horton's cephalalgia The other name for cluster headache. It is characterized by unilateral severe headache, along with autonomic symptoms like, watering from the eyes or nasal congestion. Typically, they last from 15 minutes to 3 hours and the attacks occur in clusters, lasting for weeks to months. Verapamil is successfully tried and corticosteroids and lithium can also be of some use.

Howship–Romberg phenomenon Symptom arising from a lesion in the inguinal region, referred to the knee joints, as for instance pain in a case of inguinal or obturator hernia. It occurs because the lesion presses upon the obturator nerve which ends by piercing the popliteal fascia and supplying the cruciate ligaments.

Hoyt-Spencer sign In orbital space occupying lesion, the constellation of optociliary shunt, pallor of optic disc, and visual loss. This occurs commonly in orbital nerve sheath meningioma.

Hunt and Hess scale A grading system to classify the degree of severity of subarachnoid hemorrhage, devised in 1968. It is a clinical staging and predicts the prognosis of the patient. It is divided into six categories, such as grade I, or asymptomatic with mild headache and minimal nuchal rigidity, grade 2, or moderate to severe headache, nuchal rigidity and without any neurodeficit other than cranial nerve palsy, grade 3, or drowsiness, confusion, mild focal neurodeficit, grade 4, or stupor, moderate to severe hemiparesis, grade 5, or stupor severe hemiparesis and grade 6, or coma, decerebrate posturing. The mortality increases with the increase in the grading number.

Hunter syndrome Also known as mucopolysaccharidosis II, the patients present with abdominal hernia, infections in the ear and nasal discharge. The symptoms appear at around 1 year of age. The forehead is prominent and the tongue is enlarged. The major joints are stiff with limited motion. Carpal tunnel syndrome is a complication in some cases and ivory-colored lesions in the skin is seen in the extremities. The abdomen is distended along with hepatosplenomegaly. Some of the children are mentally retarded along with attention deficit hyperactivity disorder, autism, and obsessive compulsive disorder. The urine contains an excessive amount of glycosaminoglycans. The disease is inherited in an X-linked recessive fashion.

Huntington's disease (The reader is referred to any standard textbook of neurology)

Huntington's sign When in a hemiplegic subject the patient is asked to lie supine, the lower limbs hanging by the edge of the bed, the paralyzed limb undergoes flexion at the hip and extension of the knee if he is asked to cough forcibly.

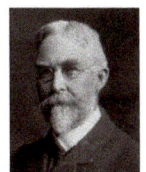

George Huntington (1850–1916, United States of America)

Hurler syndrome Also known as gargoylism or mucopolysaccharidosis type I, is of an autosomal recessive trait due to a defect in IDUA gene, mapped to chromosome 4p 16.3. There is an accumulation of the mucopolysaccharides glycosaminoglycans due to deficiency of the enzyme alpha-L-iduronidase, responsible for the degradation of mucopolysaccharides in lysosomes. There is rise of heparan sulfate and dermatan sulfate in the system. Symptoms appear in childhood. Progressive mental retardation, hepatosplenomegaly, dwarfism, coarse and bushy eyebrows, nasal discharge, retinal degeneration, and corneal clouding are the usual features. Inguinal and abdominal hernia are also sometime observed. Language is impaired due to hearing loss and enlargement of the tongue. Carpal tunnel syndrome and restricted movement in joint is sometimes an additional feature. The victims usually die by the age of 10 years from obstructive airway disease, respiratory infections or cardiac failure. Diagnosis is established by the detection of excessive urinary excretion of heparan sulfate and dermatan sulfate (Fig. H.2).

Hutchinson's pupil A clinical sign where there is dilatation of the pupil which is non-reactive to light on the side of an intracranial mass lesion following compression of the oculomotor nerve, where in stage I, parasympathetic fibers winding round the surface of the nerve are irritated, leading to pupillary constriction. Subdural and extradural hemorrhage, concussion injury to the brain or herniation of a cerebral tumor are the usual etiological factors. In stage II, these fibers are paralyzed and pupil is dilated, while the contralateral oculomotor nerve is irritated and the pupil is constricted. In stage III, the contralateral parasympathetic fibers are also paralyzed and there is bilateral dilatation of the pupil and this is known as Hutchinsonian pupil.

Hutchinson's teeth Also known as Hutchinson's incisors or mulberry teeth, these are found in congenital syphilis where the teeth are widely separated and have a crescentic notch in the biting surface. Hutchinson's teeth with interstitial keratitis and sensorineural deafness is known as Hutchinson's triad.

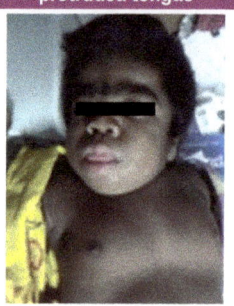

Figure H.2: Hurler syndrome. Note coarse facial features, thick bushy eyebrows, protruded tongue

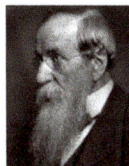

Jonathan Hutchinson
(1828–1913, United Kingdom)

Hutchinson's triad The triad of interstitial keratitis, malformed teeth or mulberry molars, and sensorineural deafness. This was described by Jonathan Hutchinson of London, often described as the greatest syphilologist of all time.

SECTION

I

Isaac syndrome Also known as neuromyotonia or continuous muscle fiber activity syndrome is a rare disorder of hyperexcitability and continuous firing of peripheral nerve axons activating the muscle fibers. The clinical picture is of muscle cramps, stiffness, slow relaxation of muscles following contraction, like myotonia, myokymia, difficulty in walking, fasciculations, intolerance to exercise, myoclonic jerks, and hyperhidrosis. The symptoms may fluctuate in severity. The condition may be acquired, hereditary, and paraneoplastic. The acquired form is the commonest one and mostly suspected to be autoimmune-mediated, caused by antibodies against neuromuscular junction. Diagnosis is established with electromyography and nerve conduction studies. Treatment with phenytoin and carbamazepine has been tried with some success. Alternatively, IVIg and plasmapheresis may be tried out.

Ishihara test A test for color blindness where blots of various colors are intermingled in a piece of paper which apparently camouflage a digital number (Fig. I.1).

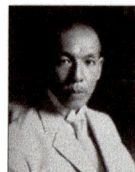

Shinobu Ishihara
(1879–1959, Japan)

Figure I.1: Ishihara's chart

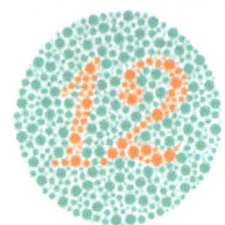

SECTION J

Jackson syndrome Paralysis of the ipsilateral 10th, 11th, and 12th cranial nerve due to a nuclear lesion. The features include, ipsilateral paralysis of soft palate, vocal cord and pharynx, ipsilateral weakness of sternomastoid and trapezius and hemiatrophy of the tongue.

Jackson's cerebellar fits Also known as *Holmes-Stewart syndrome*, it refers to a kind of posture where the head is thrown back and the spine hyperextended. The forearms and the hands are flexed, the arms kept at the sides, and the lower limbs are extended. Invariably, there is a lesion in the posterior fossa and the intracranial pressure is raised. The condition resembles decerebrate rigidity in many ways.

Jackson's law Loss of mental functions due to diseases recover in the reverse order of its evolutionary development.

Jackson's rule After an attack of epileptic fit, the nerve functions that are least developed are the least affected and recovers more rapidly than the more complex ones.

Jackson's sign During quiet respiration the movement of the paralyzed side of the chest may be greater than that of the opposite side, while in forced respiration the paralyzed side moves less than the other side.

Jackson-Mackenzie syndrome Brain stem syndrome with unilateral paralysis of soft palate, pharynx, larynx, sternocleidomastoid and trapezius muscles and hemiatrophy of the tongue.

Jacksonian seizure This refers to the phenomenon where simple partial seizure spreads from the distal part of the limb towards the ipsilateral face and is looks like a march of seizure activity. The lesion is in the primary motor cortex. The head and the eyes may turn towards the opposite side, known as adversive attack, and may lead to generalization. Consciousness is retained and there is little post-ictal confusional state. Hughlings Jackson described the condition in his first cousin, later to be his wife, who suffered from thrombosis of the superior sagittal sinus.

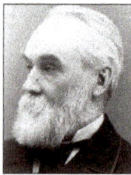

John Hughlings Jackson
(1835–1911, United Kingdom)

Jackson-Weiss syndrome A dominantly inherited form of craniosynostosis with large broad toes and fusion of the tarsal bones.

Jacobson's nerve Parasympathetic nerve fibres carried in the glossopharyngeal nerve and originating in the inferior salivary nucleus, leave the parent nerve and the petrous ganglion and travel via Jacobson's nerve to reach the otic ganglion, where the synapse.

Jacod triad Optic atrophy, total ophthalmoplegia, and trigeminal neuralgia due to a space occupying lesion in petrosphenoid space, usually from an extension of nasopharyngeal tumor.

Janz syndrome Also known as Christian Janz syndrome, it is a variety of idiopathic generalized epilepsy, manifesting between 12 to 18 years of age, characterized by attacks early in the morning on awakening. Usually, the subject does not fall but it is the objects, like the toothbrush that often drops from the hands. Muscle twitches are common in the arm, and myoclonic jerks generally precede the tonic-clonic attacks. Sleep deprivation seems to be a major trigger factor and other neurological features are usually not found. It is now a variety of ciliopathy associated with 5 causative ion channel genes, CACNB4, GABRA1, CLCN2, CABRD, and EFHC1. The gene is located in chromosome 15q14, as well as in 6p21. The EEG shows a characteristic 4–6 Hz polyspikes and slow wave discharge, usually provoked by photic stimulation and hyperventilation. Imaging studies are usually within normal limits. Sodium valproate, lamotrigine, levetiracetam, topiramate, zonisamide, and clonazepam are the preferred drugs which should be continued life-long. Carbamazepine may aggravate the symptoms and sleep deprivation must be avoided.

Jefferson's fracture Fracture of the anterior and posterior arch of the atlas bone, usually resulting from hyperextension of the neck following application of sudden brake while driving, or diving in a pool of water. Apart from pain, other features may include lateral medullary syndrome, Horner's syndrome from involvement of the sympathetic trunk, or ataxia.

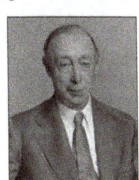

Geoffrey Jefferson
(1886–1961, United Kingdom)

Jendrassik maneuver The mechanism of recruitment of motor neurons during testing for deep tendon reflexes. It can done by pulling the closed palms together, or while testing for the upper limbs, by clenching the teeth. Recent electrophysiological experiments suggest that the facilitating effect of this maneuver on the alpha motor neurons is probably not mediated predominantly via the gamma motor loop.

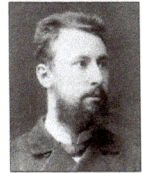

Ernö Jendrassik
(1858–1921, Hungary)

Joffroy's sign Absence of wrinkling in the forehead on upward gaze.

Jolly test The other name for repetitive nerve stimulation test for myasthenia gravis.

Joplin' neuroma A painful condition, where the digital nerve by the side of the great toe may be compressed by a scar or ill-fitting shoes.

Joubert syndrome An autosomal recessive condition where the cerebellar vermis is hypoplastic. Clinically it presents as ataxia, hyperpnoea, abnormal eye movements and hypotonia in childhood. Polydactylism, cleft lip and palate and seizures are other accompaniments. Retinitis pigmentosa is an important feature. A number of genetic mutations in a number of chromosomes have been identified and it is considered as a variety of ciliopathy. In MRI scan the classic picture is the *molar tooth sign* due to aplasia of the cerebellar vermis (Fig. J.1).

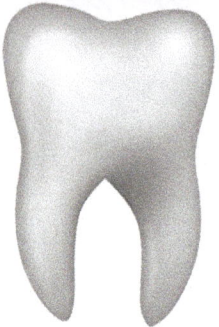
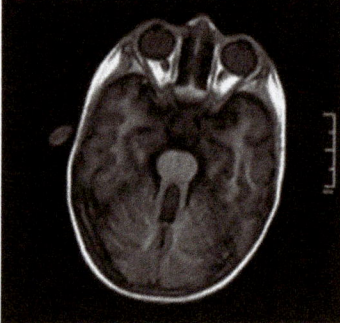

Figure J.1: Joubert syndrome. Note the molar tooth appearance of the cerebellum

SECTION K

Kallmann syndrome X-linked dominant hypogonadotrophic hypogonadism, associated with olfactory nerve agenesis and consequent anosmia. The genetic defect is at the Xp22.3 position.

Kambin's triangle A right-angled triangle over a dorsolateral lumbar disc bound by the exiting nerve root as the hypotenuse, superior border of the caudal vertebra as the base and the dura mater as the height. This triangle is used to inject epidural steroid for the amelioration of radicular pain from lumbar canal stenosis.

Kayser–Fleischer ring The golden brown ring-like structure on the Descemet's membrane of the cornea in Wilson's disease and is considered a pathognomonic sign. This is due to deposition of copper and usually starts at the upper pole, then in the lower pole, and finally the ring is completed. With neuropsychiatric manifestations in Wilson's disease the ring is almost universally present. If not visible with the naked eye, slit-lamp example can identify it. This is also seen sometime in primary biliary cirrhosis. This ring was described 8 years before Kinnier Wilson described the eponymous disease in 1910.

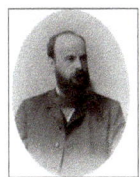

**Bruno Fleischer
(1874–1965, Germany)**

Kearns–Sayre syndrome A variety of mitochondrial disorder characterized by complete external ophthalmoplegia, retinitis pigmentosa, cardiac conduction defects, deafness, diabetes mellitus, hypoparathyroidism and some other endocrinopathies. Classically, the patients extend their neck to compensate for ptosis and obstruction to the visual field. The appearance of the consecutive optic atrophy is known as *salt-and-pepper look*. Third degree atrioventricular block and syncope is common. The condition is inherited through mitochondrial autosomal dominant or recessive transmission and there is deletions in mitochondrial DNA. The diagnosis is established by biopsy where staining the muscles with Gömöri's trichrome stain shows the blue background of normal muscles and the reddish *ragged red fibers*. Pyruvate and lactate levels are increased due to anaerobic metabolism in the CSF.

Kennedy's syndrome Also known as bulbospinal muscular atrophy, it is a neurodegenerative disorder where the motor neurons in the brain stem and the spinal cord bear the brunt of the disease. There is mutation in the androgen receptor AR gene and is inherited in an X-linked recessive manner. It is considered a disorder of androgen insensitivity. There is muscle cramp and progressive degeneration of the muscles supplied by the bulbar and spinal anterior horn cells. The onset is usually in the middle age and there is gynecomastia, erectile dysfunction, testicular atrophy and infertility. There is increase in the CAG trinucleotide repeats and this is the first disease where repeat expansions were first observed.

Kernig's sign A sign of meningeal irritation. When the lower limb is flexed at 90 degrees at the hip and the examiner tries to extend the knee joint, pain is felt at the back, due to spasm in the hamstring muscles. This is a classic bedside test to diagnose meningitis and subarachnoid hemorrhage, along with neck stiffness.

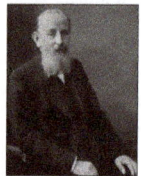

Woldemer Kernig (1840–1917, Russia)

Kernohan's notch phenomenon The free margin of the tentorium cerebelli is close to the cerebral peduncle which carries the corticospinal tract from the ipsilateral side in its middle two-thirds. In case of a large space-occupying lesion of the opposite side, the cerebral peduncle is pushed against the free edge of the tentorium cerebelli which produces a visible notch on its surface. This produces pyramidal tract sign in the ipsilateral side of the lesion. Thus, this is an example of a false localizing sign and an ipsilateral cerebral event. It is also known as *Kernohan-Woltman sign*.

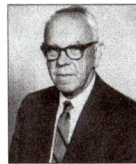

James Watson Kernohan (1896–1981, United states of America)

Kestenbaum's sign It refers to the number of arterioles crossing the optic disc in the retina. If the number is less than 5, it indicates primary optic atrophy.

Kiloh-Nevin syndrome The other name for anterior interosseous nerve syndrome, where a fibrous band constricts it, or an accessory head of the flexor pollicis longus muscle, known as *Gantzer's muscle*, traps it.

Kinsbourne disease Opso-clonus-myoclonus syndrome in children. It usually follows neuroblastoma as paraneoplastic syndrome, exanthematous fever or vaccination.

Kirsch reflex The other name for auriculopalpebral reflex. The eyes close involuntarily in response to a loud sound.

Kjellin's syndrome A hereditary, autosomal recessive, neuro-ophthalmologic syndrome characterized by spastic paraplegia, dementia, dysarthria, corpus callosal atrophy and dystrophy of the posterior pole of the ocular fundus.

Klaus height index The distance between the tip of the dens and the tuberculum torcula line. Normally it is from 40–41 mm. This is reduced in basilar invagination.

Kleine–Levin syndrome A rare disorder that primarily affects adolescent males. It is characterized by recurring but reversible periods of excessive sleep, up to 20 hours per day. The symptoms last for a few days to few weeks and the onset is abrupt. Classically, there is hyperphagia, irritability, childishness and hypersexuality. Depression is often a predominant feature. Patients are characteristically amnestic about the event when they are normal. Viral infections may trigger the attack and herpes zoster, influenza A, Epstein–Barr, varicella, etc. have been implicated. Lesion in the hypothalamus and thalamus, parts of the brain that govern appetite and sleep is considered a possibility and an imbalance in serotonin and dopamine activity could be the biochemical abnormality. Many researchers feel that the demon character *Kumbhakarna* in the epic *The Ramayana* was a victim of Kleine-Levin syndrome.

Klippel–Feil syndrome There is congenital fusion of any two of the cervical vertebrae, leading the limitation in nuchal movement, short neck and low hair line. It is often associated with craniovertebral anomalies and Arnold–Chiari malformation. It may be transmitted as an autosomal dominant or recessive condition and mutation in GDF6 and GDF3 have been identified. Incidentally, the dominant variety presents with fusion in C2 and C3 vertebrae, while in the recessive variety the fusion is between C5 and C6 vertebrae. Another autosomal dominant form mapped on locus 8q22.2, known as Klippel–Feil syndrome with laryngeal malformation has been identified.

Klippel–Trénaunay-Weber syndrome Classically, a triad of vascular malformations of the capillary, venous and lymphatic vessels, varicosities in unusual anatomical locations and unilateral soft tissue and skeletal hypertrophy, usually in the lower extremities, leading to local gigantism. There is some evidence that translocation at 8q22.3 gene can be an association, while others have linked it to the VG5Q gene.

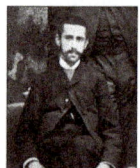

Maurice Klippel (1858–1942, France)

Klüver–Bucy syndrome

A condition characterized by hyperphagia, visual agnosia, restlessness, hyperorality, over-attentiveness to visual stimuli, hypersexuality, and loss of ability to learn new skills. It happens classically in bilateral temporal lobe damage following encephalitis, head injury, etc.

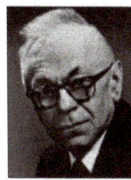

Heinrich Klüver (1897–1979, United states of America)

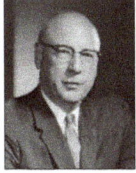

Paul Bucy (1904–1992, United states of America)

Kocher–Debré-Sémalaigne syndrome

A complication of hypothyroidism in infancy, where there is gross hypertrophy of the calf muscles. When such features are present in adulthood it is known as *Hoffman's syndrome*.

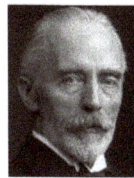

Emil Theodor Kocher (1841–1917, Switzerland)

Kohs block design test A performance test where the subject is given 16 colored cubes and he has to replicate the patterns on a series of test cards. The test is grossly affected in persons with right hemispheric lesion.

Köllner's rule Red and green differentiation difficulty is a common feature of primary optic atrophy, while in retinochoroidal illnesses the difficulty is more in discriminating yellow from blue colour.

Korsakoff's syndrome A syndrome of combined Wernicke's encephalopathy and Korsakoff's psychosis. It manifests initially as an acute encephalopathic picture, followed by psychotic features in chronic and malnourished abusers of alcohol. Wernicke's encephalopathy is caused by thiamine deficiency and consists of opthalmoplegia, confusion and ataxia of gait. Among the extraocular muscles, lateral rectus is most commonly involved and ataxia results from involvement of the cerebellum, as well as the vestibular system. Hypotension, hypothermia and seizures are the terminal manifestations. Korsakoff's syndrome is characterized by severe amnesia without intellectual decline. The nature of the amnesia is mostly anterograde, but it can be retrograde as well. Aphasia, apraxia, agnosia, confabulation, and problems in executive functions are associated features.

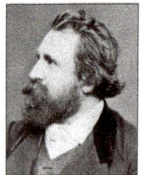

Sergei Sergeievich Korsakoff
(1853–1900, Russia)

Kozhevnikov-Rasmussen syndrome The other name for epilepsy partialis continua. This is a variety of partial epilepsy, often accompanied by Jacksonian march of events and Todd's palsy. This is usually caused by a focal congenital or acquired lesion in the brain.

Theodore Brown Rasmussen
(1910–2002)

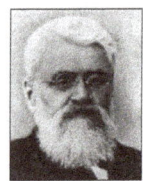

Aleksei Kozhevnikov
(1836–1902, Russia)

Krabbe's disease Also known as globoid cell leukodystrophy, it occurs in infancy and manifests as seizures, irritability, mental slowness and muscular weakness. Deafness, spasticity, optic atrophy and optic nerve enlargement are other features. It is inherited as an autosomal recessive disorder and the mutation is in the GALC gene in chromosome 14q31. The enzyme deficient is galactosylceramidase.

Krause's end bulb Cutaneous receptors sensitive to cold feeling.

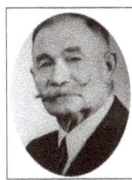

Johann Friedrich Wilhelm Krause (1833–1910, Germany)

Kufs disease A condition characterized under the rubric of neuronal ceroid lipofuscinoses. The patients present with visual problems, cognitive dysfunction, seizures, myoclonic epilepsy and ataxia. The pathology is due to the buildup of keratin in the skin.

Kugelberg-Welander disease The other name for spinal muscular atrophy type 3. It presents with muscular weakness, areflexia, wasting, fasciculations, and scoliosis. It is an autosomal recessive condition and the mutation is in the SMA1 gene in chromosome 5q13. It is diagnosed with electromyography and biopsy.

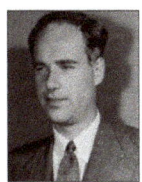

Eric Klas Hendrik Kugelberg (1913–1983, Sweden)

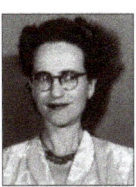

Lisa Welander (1909–2001, Sweden)

Kurtzke Expanded Disability Status Scale A scale devised to measure the status of disability of subjects with multiple sclerosis. It provides a total scale ranging from 0 to 10 in increasing order of severity. Levels 1 to 4.5 refer to disability of lesser intensity with high ambulatory capability, while that from 5 to

9.5 indicates lesser ambulation. In addition, it provided eight subscale measurements, called Functional System Score on the basis of pyramidal, cerebellar, brainstem, sensory, bowel and bladder, visual, mental and other functions.

Labbé's vein Also known as the inferior anastomotic vein, it is a part of superficial venous system of the brain. It is the largest channel crossing across temporal lobe between the Sylvian fissure and the transverse sinus and connects the superior middle cerebral vein to the transverse sinus.

Lafora body disease A fatal disease of autosomal recessive inheritance where characteristic inclusion bodies known as *Lafora bodies* are found in the cytoplasm of the liver, heart, skin and muscles. It is now considered a glycogen metabolism disorder. The onset is usually in adolescence and the presenting features are seizures, myoclonus ataxia and rapidly progressive dementia. There is mutation in the EPM2A, EPM2B, and NHLRC1 genes, which code for the protein laforin, malin, and ubiquitin ligase, respectively. The chromosome implicated is 6p23-27. The diagnosis is established by cutaneous biopsy of the sweat glands from the axilla, which on PAS stain, demonstrate the Lafora bodies.

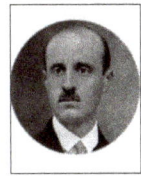

Gonzalo Rodríguez Lafora (1886–1971, Spain)

Laing myopathy A variety of distal myopathy of childhood. There is weakness in certain muscles in the feet and ankles which leads to tightening of the tendoachilis, an inability to lift the big toe, and a high-steppage gait. Later, there is weakness in muscles of the hands and wrists which makes lifting the fingers, particularly the third and the fourth digit, difficult. Tremor in the hands is a common symptom. Later, there is weakness in neck and facial muscles and even later, it extends to other muscles in the body as well. Life expectancy is usually within normal limits. The disease is inherited as an autosomal recessive trait and there is mutation in the MYH7 gene, leading to deficiency in the production of type II myosin and reduced contractility of the muscles. In spite of the fact that myosin is found abundantly in cardiac muscles, the heart remains unaffected in this condition.

Lambert's sign Transient improvement of ptosis in Lambert–Eaton syndrome on sustained upgaze. This is how it can be differentiated from myasthenia gravis, where ptosis is aggravated.

Lance–Adams syndrome Post hypoxic action myoclonus occurring days to weeks after the patient regains consciousness following cardiopulmonary resuscitation. Electroencephalography shows diffuse slowing. Sodium valproate, clonazepam, levetiracetam, piracetam, zonisamide, and 5-hydroxytryptophan have all been used in order to reduce the severity of myoclonus. Recently, perampanel, a selective, noncompetitive, α-amino-3-hydroxy-5-methyl-4-isoxazolepropionic acid receptor antagonist, approved for the management of epilepsy, has been used with some success.

Landau–Kleffner syndrome Also known as acquired epileptic aphasia, this rare variety of epileptic syndrome in childhood manifests itself as sudden or gradual onset aphasia and an abnormal EEG pattern. It typically occurs between 3 and 7 years of age and the affected children lose their language skill. Seizures may occur while others may exhibit only EEG changes, including electrographic status epilepticus. Auditory verbal agnosia is the commonest problem in speech where the subjects fail to lateralize the sound and familiar sounds may be registered as alien. Prognostically, subjects who manifest signs early and have nocturnal seizures, have poorer outcome. Behavioral and other neuropsychiatric complications are also common in the form of hyperactivity, reduced attention span, aggression and anxiety and it is generally said that these result from the speech defect. The yield in EEG is maximum after overnight recording. PET scan shows hypometabolism in both the temporal lobes. Anticonvulsants, corticosteroids and ACTH have been used with success. Multiple subpial resection is surgical mode of a therapy which can be employed.

Landry–Guillain–Barré–Strohl syndrome

A few words about the history of the nomenclature shall not be out of place. It is said that the original paper on this condition was written by Georges Guillain, Alexandre Barré, and André Strohl in 1916. Octave Landry's name was added to it later and Guillain remarked that it only added to the nosological confusion. Interestingly, Strohl's name has somewhat been forgotten with the passage of time. (The reader is referred to any standard textbook of neurology)

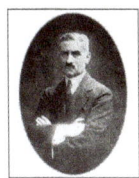

**Georges Guillain
(1876–1961, France)**

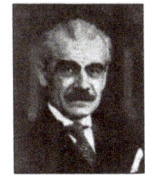

**Jean Alexandre Barré
(1880–1967, France)**

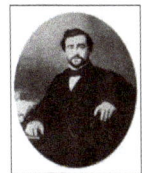

**Octave Landry
(1826–1865, France)**

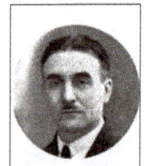

André Strohl
(1887–1977, France)

Lasègue's disease The other name for paranoia.

Lasègue's sign The other name for straight leg raising sign. With the patient lying supine, he or she is asked to raise it. In case of lumbar disc herniation, pain is felt due to impingement on the lumbar nerve roots by the herniated nucleus pulposus of the intervertebral disc through the ruptured annulus fibrosus. The story goes that Lasègue thought of this sign when he saw his son-in-law tuning a violin string stretching over the white piece of ivory which supports the strings. He immediately surmised that stretching the sciatic nerve might cause pain if it is compressed by the prolapsed disc. In lumbar root compression, flexion of the hip is painful when the knee is extended, but not when the knee is flexed.

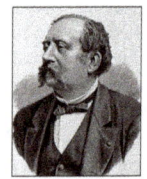

Ernest-Charles Lasègue
(1816–1883, France)

Lasègue-Falret syndrome Association psychosis syndrome, or *'folie à deux'*, where a delusional belief or hallucinatory feeling is transmitted from one individual to another.

Lazarus sign A sign of brain death, where movements like, flexion of the upper limbs, adduction of the shoulders, raising of the arms, and even crossing of the hands can be observed. These are presumably due to intact autonomous spinal reflex, which are now released from supraspinal cortical inhibitory influence. Obviously, this refers to the story from Gospel of John, where Martha, a lady, took his deceased brother Lazarus after 4 days to Jesus

Christ and Christ said, '*Lazarus, come forth*' and Lazarus came alive.

Leber's optic atrophy A mitochondrial disease inherited maternally, where there is degeneration of the ganglion cells of the retina and their axons, leading to progressive visual loss. It presents with vision loss due to optic atrophy, first in one eye and weeks to months later, the other eye is involved. The onset is in the young age. Point mutations in MT-ND1, 4 and 6 genes lead to this condition.

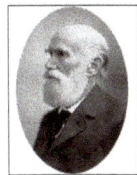

Theodor Leber
(1840–1917, Germany)

Leigh's disease An inherited neurometabolic disease affecting the central nervous system. The symptoms appear in early childhood leading to death in a few years. Infection is often a triggering factor and the disease may be episodic or progressive with developmental delay. The affected children cry much more than what is usual. Seizures, hypotonia, dystonia, ataxia, ophthalmoparesis and nystagmus are the usual neurological manifestations. Some children suffer from hypertrophic cardiomyopathy and ventricular septal defect. Hypertrichosis is common and most of the children die of respiratory failure. Mutations occur in mitochondrial DNA and over 30 genes have been described. Excessive amount of lactate is observed in urine, cerebrospinal fluid and blood. MRI in T2 image shows hyperintensity in brainstem, medulla and classically in putamen.

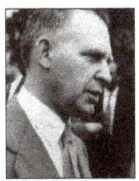

Denis Archibald Leigh
(1916–1998, United Kingdom)

Lennox–Gastaut syndrome A childhood onset epileptic syndrome carrying grave prognosis and appearing mostly in the first decade of life. It is characterized by the triad of frequent and multiple seizure types, a typical EEG picture of less than 2.5 Hz slow spike and slow wave activity, best brought out with under-provocative measures, and severe intellectual impairment. Nocturnal tonic seizure is the commonest variety, though myoclonic, atonic, atypical absence, partial and generalized seizures are also not uncommon. Nonconvulsive seizures are also seen in many patients. Behavioral disorders and psychomotor problems are also frequent. Majority of the cases are secondary and in a number of cases it is the termination of West syndrome, and encephalopathy, tuberous sclerosis, hereditary metabolic disorders, encephalitis, meningitis, ischemic-hypoxic brain damage are the precipitating factors. Idiopathic cases have better prognosis. Mutation in CHD2, GABRB3, ALG13 and SCN2A genes have been reported. Felbamate, a drug known to cause hypoplastic anemia has been found effective, along with lamotrigine, topiramate and rufinamide. Interestingly, nitrazepam may paradoxically worsen the condition. Ketogenic diet is also an alternative as is intravenous immunoglobulin. In refractory cases, corpus callosotomy and vagal nerve stimulation can be undertaken.

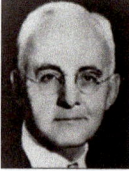

William Gordon Lennox (1884–1960, United States of America)

Leo's spreading depression
A wave of electrophysiological hyperactivity, followed by a period of inhibition, observed in migrainous aura and it often predicts an impending cerebrovascular accident.

Leri's band A congenital fibrous or fatty band that stretches across the pelvis and compresses upon the cauda equina and leads to cauda equina syndrome.

Lesch–Nyhan syndrome

A rare X-linked metabolic disorder of purine metabolism caused by mutation in HPRT gene due to deficiency in the enzyme hypoxanthine-guanine phophoribosyl transferase. This leads to accumulation of huge amounts of uric acid in the body. The neurological signs include moderate intellectual decline, self-mutilation, like obsessive lip and nail biting, accompanied with severe gouty arthritis. Facial grimacing and repetitive movements of the upper and lower extremities are common neurological features. Megaloblastic anemia is an accompaniment since lack of the enzyme leads to improper utilization of vitamin B12.

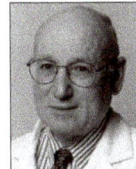

Michael Lesch (1939–2008, United States of America)

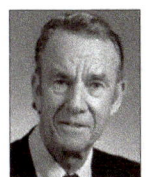

William Nyhan (1926–till date, United States of America)

Lewy body Abnormal aggregates of proteins, found in the neurons in Parkinson's disease, diffuse Lewy body disease, multiple system atrophy, and sometimes in amyotrophic lateral sclerosis and even, in normal individuals. They are intracytoplasmic eosinophilic spherical inclusion bodies made of alpha-synuclein, found predominantly in the substantia nigra, but also in the cortex at a later stage of the disease. Additionally, ubiquitin, neurofilament protein, alpha B crystalline and tau proteins may also be present. Initially, Lewy did not attach much attention to these structure and it was left to Konstantin Nikolaevitch Tretiakoff to find out their significance and he named these as *corps de Lewy*.

Lewy neurites Abnormal neurites, axons or dendrites from a neuron, which contain granular materials and abnormal alpha-synuclein filaments as are found in Lewy bodies. These are features of diseases designated as alpha-synucleinopathies.

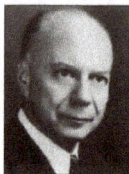

Friedrich Heinrich Lewy (1885–1950, United States of America)

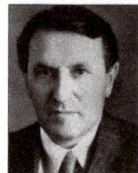

Konstantin Tretiakoff (1892–1958, Russia)

Leyden–Möebius dystrophy A variety of limb girdle muscular dystrophy, of both autosomal dominant and recessive inheritance, appearing in childhood or adolescence with predilection for both the sexes. It is characterized by weakness, symmetrical wasting of the pelvic and shoulder girdle muscles with sparing of facial muscles. No muscle hypertrophy, cardiac conduction defect or cardiomyopathy, and mental retardation is observed.

Lhermitte's sign Sudden flexion of the neck produces an electric shock like sensation in conditions where the posterior column is compromised. Though classically described in multiple sclerosis, where plaques damage the column, it may be positive in cervical spondylotic myelopathy. This is also known as *Barber Chair sign,* indicating the head posture when the barber trims the hair at the back of the head, which may trigger the symptom. The condition is also known as *Lhermitte-Lévy syndrome*.

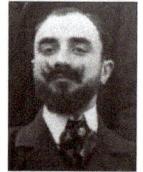

Jacques Jean Lhermitte (1877–1959, France)

Liddell-Sherrington reflex
Tonic contraction of muscles occurs in response to its being stretched.

Lissauer tract Also known as the posterolateral tract, it is a small group of nerve fiber situated near the tip of the dorsal cord at the point of entry of the sensory nerve roots and it is most prominent in the cervical cord. It contains centrally projecting axons from the dorsal root ganglia cells which carry crude touch and pressure sensation. These axons penetrate the gray matter of the dorsal horn and synapse with the second order neurons in substantia gelatinosa or the nucleus proprius. These neurons now send their axons to the other half of the spinal cord, where they constitute the lateral spinothalamic tract, which in turn synapse in the ventral posterolateral nucleus of the thalamus. The third order neurons now terminate in the post central gyrus, completing the sensory system. In occlusion of the anterior spinal artery it is the only tract spared along with the posterior column, whereas they are involved in subacute combined degeneration of the spinal cord.

Little's disease Also known as spastic diplegia, it is a form of cerebral palsy where there is spasticity, hypertonia and hyperreflexia in the lower limbs. While walking, the limbs tend to cross each other and this is known as *scissors gait*. Baclofen, tolperisone, botulinum toxin, physiotherapy, and selective posterior rhizotomy can lead to some improvement.

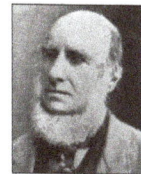

William John Little
(1810–1894, United Kingdom)

Locock's bromide Sir Charles Locock first introduced the use of bromide for the management of epilepsy. He published his observations in *The Lancet* in 1857. Incidentally, he was an obstetrician and was appointed as the first ever obstetrician to

Queen Victoria in 1840. He supervised the birth of all her nine children from 1840 to 1857.

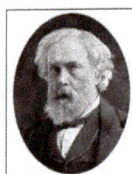

**Sir Charles Locock
(1799–1875, United Kingdom)**

Looser zone Transverse lines in X-ray in bones like inferior ramus of the pubis, proximal femur or tibia, ribs etc. in conditions like, osteomalacia, rickets, hyperthyroidism, Paget's disease, osteogenesis imperfecta, etc. These lines do not involve the entire breadth of the bone and is only partial and therefore, often known as *pseudofractures*. It is postulated that these are found at the site where the nutrient artery enters the bone and in these conditions where the bone density is reduced, their pulsation leads to this appearance. Most of these conditions present with features of proximal myopathy, positive Gower's sign, etc (Fig. L.1).

Figure L.1: Looser zone

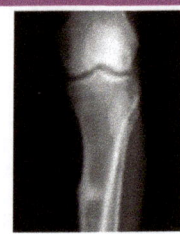

Lou Gehrig's disease The other name for amyotrophic lateral sclerosis. Lou Gehrig himself suffered from it and is widely regarded as an outstanding baseball player from USA.

Louis–Bar syndrome The other old name for ataxia telangiectasia. This is a rare autosomal recessive disorder characterized by cerebellar ataxia and scleral telangiectasia. The affected children have difficulty in moving their eyes from one place to another, which suggests oculomotor apraxia. Additionally, the children suffer from chronic sinu-pulmonary infections, vitiligo, lymphoma, leukemia and progeria. High level of alpha-fetoprotein is found in the blood. The defect is located on chromosome 11q22.3

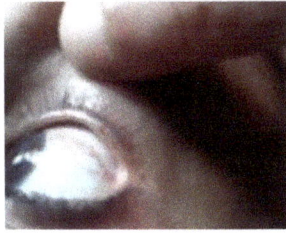

Figure L.2: Louis–Bar syndrome showing conjunctival telangiectasia

and is caused by a defect in ATM gene (Fig. L.2).

Lowe syndrome Also known as oculocerebrorenal syndrome, it is a rare X-linked recessive disorder, characterized by cataracts, hypotonia, intellectual underdevelopment, proximal tubular acidosis, aminoaciduria and proteinuria. Some consider this disorder as a variety of Fanconi syndrome. The condition is caused by mutation in the OCRL1 gene.

Luria test Also known as the fist-palm-edge test, it asks the subject to tap the table with the fist, then the palm, and finally the edge quickly in succession, after being instructed and taught to do so. The examiner observes whether the subject can do it without mistakes. This is one of the components of the FAB, or the Frontal Lobe Assessment Battery test. The other test in the name of Luria is the *Graphomotor test,* where the subject is instructed to draw a series of loops or spirals, or cursive Ms and Ns. This test is routinely performed in the assessment of cognitive function.

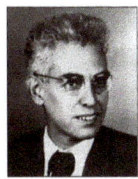

Alexander Luria
(1902–1977, Russia)

Luschka foramen The two lateral foramina on the roof of the 4th ventricle through which cerebrospinal fluid escapes to the subarachnoid space.

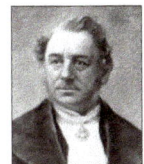

Hubert von Luschka
(1820–1875, Germany)

Luys nucleus Also known as corpus luysi, it is the other name for the subthalamic nucleus, the pea-shaped structures looking up and out ventral to the thalami and dorsal to the substantia nigra. In recent times, it has assumed importance since it is the target for deep brain stimulation for the management of the intractable late complications like, dyskinesia and on-off phenomenon with levodopa therapy.

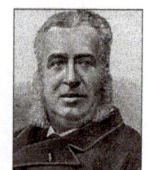

Jules Bernard Luys (1828–1897, France)

SECTION M

Macewen's sign A sign to diagnose childhood hydrocephalus. Tapping the skull near the junction of the frontal, temporal and parietal bones shall produce a *cracked pot sound*, indicating separated sutures resulting from raised intracranial pressure.

Madelung's disease A syndrome of peripheral neuropathy associated with multiple lipomas. Usually, there is history of alcohol abuse.

Magendie's foramen The central foramen in the roof of the 4th ventricle through which cerebrospinal fluid escapes into the subarachnoid space.

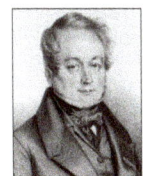

**François Magendie
(1783–1855, France)**

Magnan's symptom A peculiar sensation, as if insects are crawling beneath the skin. Also known as cocaine bugs, this is found in cocaine intoxication. It was described by Valentin Magnan, an outstanding psychiatrist from France in his time. He did remarkable works on the evils of alcohol.

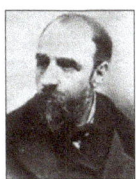

**Valentin Magnan
(1835–1916, France)**

Mallory stain A method of demonstrating glial fibers under the microscope. It uses mercuric chloride, phosphotungstic acid, and alcohol. Muscle fibers, myelin and glial cells stain blue, while collagen fibers stain brown.

Marburg multiple sclerosis

Also known as acute fulminant multiple sclerosis, it is considered by some authorities as a variant of multiple sclerosis, while others feel that it is a separate entity. Others again consider it as the other name for tumefactive multiple sclerosis. It is a relentlessly progressive disorder with grave prognosis within 2 years.

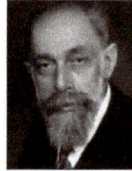

Otto Marburg
(1874–1948, Austria)

Marchiafava–Bignami syndrome A progressive neurological disease as a complication of alcoholism, characterized by demyelination of the corpus callosum and necrosis and subsequent atrophy. Clinically, motor or cognitive disturbances, disconnection syndromes and seizures are the usual manifestations. It is caused by deficiencies of the vitamin B group.

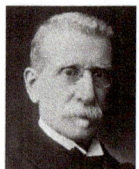

Ettore Marchiafava
(1847–1935, Italy)

Marcus Gunn phenomenon

This condition is also known as *jaw-winking phenomenon*. Rhythmic upward elevation of the upper eyelid is associated with jaw opening or closing, and usually it is unilateral. It is a variety of congenital synkinesis between oculomotor nerve, supplying levator palpebrae superioris and the trigeminal nerve, supplying the pterygoids or masseter. It is postulated that this syndrome is due to an exaggeration of a weak physiological cocontraction between muscles supplied by the two nerves resulting from a congenital lesion in the brain stem nuclei. *Inverse Marcus Gunn phenomenon* refers to the condition where there is drooping of the eyelid on opening the jaw. More often than not, it is an acquired phenomenon.

Marcus Gunn pupil Also known as relative afferent pupillary defect, the pupil is tested by flashing light on one pupil and swinging it to the other pupil after 3 seconds. Normally, light directed on any normal pupil will produce direct and consensual light reflexes of equal response. However, in demyelinating lesion of one eye, like retrobulbar neuritis, the response evoked by flashing light into that eye will be lesser than what will be produced if light is shown in the normal eye. This indicates only partial lesion in the optic nerve since in complete lesion, no response shall be evoked on stimulation by light.

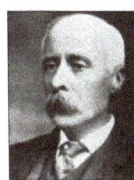

Robert Marcus Gunn
(1850–1909, United Kingdom)

Marie's ataxia The other name for autosomal dominant cerebellar ataxias.

Marie's crossed adduction reflex Crossed, contralateral, adductor reflex.

Marie's paper test A test of comprehension, where the subject is given a piece of paper and asked to tear it into four parts, place one on the table, offer one to the examiner to keep the remaining two pieces for himself. An affected subject shall commit some error somewhere.

Marie-Foix retraction sign In patients with pyramidal tract lesion, where there is flexion of hip and knee on pressure over the toes.

Marie-Foix syndrome Unilateral cerebellar ataxia with contralateral hemiparesis and thermoanalgesia resulting from infarction of rostral pontine region.

Marie-Foix-Alajouanine syndrome Cerebellar ataxia of old age, frequently due to alcohol abuse.

Marie-Sée syndrome The other name for idiopathic intracranial hypertension following ingestion of large dose of vitamin A.

Marie-Strümpell disease The other name for ankylosing spondylitis.

Marie-Strümpell encephalitis
The other name for acute infantile hemiplegia.

Marinacci anastomosis
An abnormal communication between the ulnar and the median nerve in the palm. It resembles Martin-Gruber anastomosis, which is the median and the ulnar nerve anastomosis. However, incidence of Marinacci anastomosis is much less.

Marinesco hand sign
Cold, livid and edematous hand in syringomyelia with sausage-like fingers. This results from sympathetic irritation.

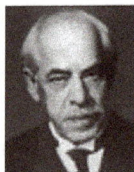

Gheorghe Marinesco
(1863–1938, Romania)

Markesbery-Griggs myopathy
A variety of distal myopathy where the anterior compartment of the legs is wasted. It is a slowly progressive disease which starts after the age of 35. The mutation is in TTN gene and the abnormal protein is known as titin.

Maroteaux-Lamy syndrome
Also known as mucopolysaccharoidosis VI, the symptoms are corneal clouding like many of the related conditions, deafness, dural thickening and pain. The trunk is short, stance crouched and joint movement restricted with contracture. The tongue is large and protruded, facial bones deformed, abdomen is protruded with umbilical and inguinal hernia, and cardiac valvular dysfunctions. The condition is inherited in an autosomal recessive pattern and there are mutations in the ARSB gene which provides the instruction for the production of the enzyme arylsulfatase B, which is deficient in this disease. Arylsulfatase B helps in the breakdown of large sugar molecules called glycosaminoglycans and there is accumulation of glycosaminoglycans in the lysosomes with consequent increase in the size of the cells leading to organomegaly, cellular inflammation and death. Galsulfase, an enzyme that corrects the underlying deficiency has shown some improvement. Currently, this agent, along with

Figure M.1: Maroteaux-Lamy syndrome. Note dysmorphic facial features, swollen knees, protruded tongue and contracture in the joints of the fingers

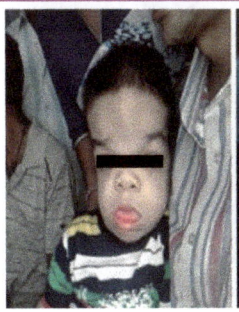
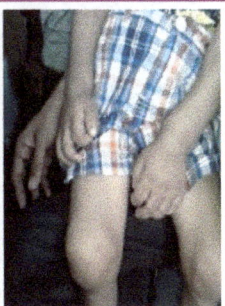

nusenersin, a drug used for the management of SMA type I are the two most expensive drugs in the world (Fig. M.1).

Marsden's long latency (M1, M2, M3, loop)

The stretch reflex is supposed to have a cortical component where on stretching a muscle, the afferent impulse travels up the spinal cord to the motor cortex and returns to the spinal efferent neurons and results in a separate reflex of long latency, apart from the classical spinal monosynaptic stretch reflex. While recording the stretch reflex, the latencies are recorded. The first M1 is the short involuntary monosynaptic spinal stretch reflex involving primary afferents, the second M2 represents the long transcortical loop latency, while the third M3 represents the latency for a voluntary response mediated by the cerebellum. The name M1, M2, and M3 has been assigned to C David Marsden, Pat Merton and HB Morton for their stupendous work on stretch reflex in the early 1970s.

Marsden's triple cocktail

The combination of an anticholinergic, tetrabenazine, and pimozide for the management of myoclonic dystonia.

Marsden's triple... Martin-Amat syndrome

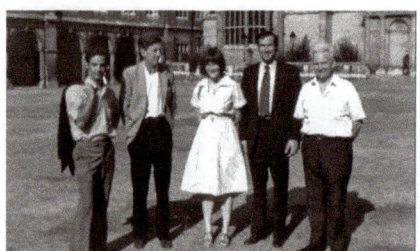

The '3 Ms' at the Centenary Meeting of the Physiological Society in Trinity College, Cambridge in 1976. David Marsden is at the extreme left, followed by Pat Merton, Jane Adam, one of Marsden's first two PhD students, Mark Hallett, Marsden's fellow at King's College, London, who worked on the electrophysiology of Myoclonus, and Bert Morton. (*Courtesy*, Professor Mark Hallett, Bethesda, USA)

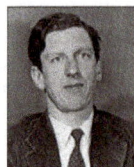

Patrick Anthony Merton
(1920–2000. United Kingdom)

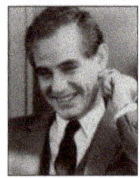

C David Marsden
(1938–1998, United Kingdom)

Martin Amat sign Following Bell's palsy, the patient may close the eyes while smiling. This is due to aberrant synkinesis following recovery of the damaged facial nerve.

Martin-Amat syndrome Involuntary closure of one eye when patients with lower motor facial palsy open their mouth. This is due to an aberrant synkinesis between the oculomotor nerve supplying levator palpebrae superioris, and the mandibular division of the trigeminal nerve, supplying the lateral pterygoid muscles, which help in opening the jaw.

Martin-Gruber anastomosis

This is the most commonly encountered anomaly of communication between two peripheral nerves. Here, motor fibers from the median nerve, destined to supply the superficial forearm muscles, the anterior interosseous nerve, or directly from the median nerve, cross, usually in the mid-forearm, to join the ulnar nerve. These fibers then run along with the ulnar nerve to innervate the first dorsal interosseous, (the commonest muscle), abductor digiti minimi, adductor pollicis, deep head of flexor pollicis brevis, or a combination of these muscles. This anomalous innervation is diagnosed during nerve conduction studies of the upper limb, where stimulating the ulnar nerve at the wrist or below the elbow, and recording the response from the abductor digiti minimi, the first muscle to be affected in lesions of the ulnar nerve, results in a pseudoconduction block, while stimulating the median nerve proximally the compound muscle action potential is recorded from the abductor digiti minimi. In one cadaveric study, this anomaly was found to be in the range of 29% of subjects.

Mayer-Gross closing-in phenomenon
In diffuse cortical damage, when a subject is asked to copy a figure, they draw either too close to the original test material, or sometime superimpose their own drawing on the sample supplied.

McArdle sign
Increase in weakness in the limbs in flexion of the neck, and its subsequent relief on extension in demyelinating pathology of the spinal cord. It is suggested that ischemia increases on flexion of the neck.

McArdle syndrome
Glycogen storage disease type V, caused by myophosphorylase deficiency. A disorder of childhood, it is characterized by muscle pain, exercise intolerance, fatigability, muscle cramps and myoglobinuria following rhabdomyolysis. Some patients experience the '*second wind phenomenon*', where the patient tolerates exercise better if he or she walks or rides a bicycle for some time. It is an autosomal recessive disease and the chromosomal locus is at 11q13.

McDonald criteria A criteria for the diagnosis of multiple sclerosis devised by William Ian McDonald of Queen Square, London in 2001 while directing an international panel of experts on behalf of the National Multiple Sclerosis Society of America and it replaced the earlier practiced Poser criteria, or the even older Schumacher criteria. It appreciates the criterion advanced by Charles Poser of Harvard that there must be dissemination of lesions in space and time, but discourages terms like, clinically definite, or possible multiple sclerosis. On the contrary, the suggestion is either possible or not multiple sclerosis. This criteria, accepted the role of MRI as surrogate marker for the spread of the disease in space and time.

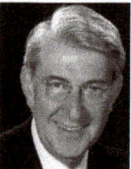

William Ian McDonald
(1933–2006, United Kingdom)

McGregor line An imaginary line in the lateral view of the skull, connecting the posterior edge of the hard palate to the most caudal point of the occipital protuberance. In basilar invagination, the tip of the odontoid process lies more than 4.5 mm above this line.

McLeod syndrome Also known as choreoacanthocytosis, this X-linked autosomal recessive disease occurs almost exclusively in males. They present with choreiform movements, myoclonic jerks, and dystonia of the face and throat which leads to chocking and spillage of food from the mouth. Myopathy, peripheral neuropathy, depression, bipolar disorders, or obsessive-compulsive traits are commonly associated with this condition. Dilated cardiomyopathy and cardiac dysrhythmias often predispose to sudden death. Acanthocytes are often seen in the peripheral blood film. Mutation is seen in the *XK* gene and *Kelly antigen* is often found in red blood corpuscles.

McRae's line An imaginary line in the lateral view of the skull connecting the basion and the opisthion. Normally, the tip of the odontoid process is 5 mm below this line and if it is above the line, it indicates basilar invagination.

Meige's syndrome A condition characterized by involuntary and often forceful contractions of the muscles of the jaw and tongue or oromandibular dystonia and involuntary muscle spasms and contractions of the muscles around the eyes or blepharospasm. Anticholinergics, tetrabenazine, baclofen etc., may be tried but most subjects require botulinum toxin therapy eventually. The condition is also known as *Brueghel's syndrome*.

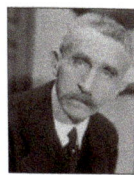

Henri Meige
(1866–1940, France)

Meissner's corpuscles Sensory receptors in the skin, sensitive to touch.

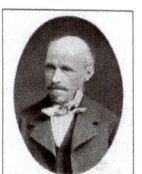

Georg Meissner
(1829–1905, Germany)

Melkersson–Rosenthal syndrome The combination of recurrent facial palsy, blubbery lips, and trident tongue. It may be a familial condition. The onset is in adolescence and following recurrent attacks the changes may be permanent. Certain ethnic groups in Bolivia seem to be prone to the condition and it may be the forerunner of Crohn's disease and sarcoidosis.

Melzack-Torgerson pain index A scale for rating pain by self-report questionnaire that describes the quality and intensity of pain.

Ménière's disease A disease of the inner year where the chief symptoms are vertigo, hearing loss, a sense of fullness in the year, and vomiting, each episode lasting from 20 minutes to 1 hour. It is believed that the symptoms appear due to collection of endolymphatic fluid in the labyrinth of the inner ear. The lesion is classically unilateral to start with and with time the problems tend to become permanent. The definite diagnostic criteria include, audiometrically documented low to medium frequency sensorineural deafness on at least one episode, fluctuating aural symptoms of tinnitus in the affected ear and not better explained by any other vestibular pathology. Both genetic and environmental factors are implicated in the pathogenesis. Treatment consists in extremely low dose of sodium in diet, anti-emetics, vestibular sedatives like, betahistine, cinnarizine, dimenhydrinate, loop diuretics like furosemide, or torsemide in order to reduce labyrinthine fluid content, injection of intraaural aminoglycoside like, gentamicin and destroying the labyrinthine system chemically, and by surgical interventions like, decompression of the endolymphatic sac or vestibular neurectomy.

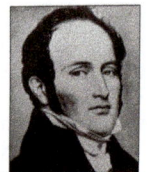

Prosper Ménière (1799–1862, France)

Menkes kinky hair disease

An X-linked recessive disease of unusually kinked hair due to copper deficiency. The neurological signs are generalized seizures, mental retardation, corpus callosal agenesis, and demyelination. A combination of this condition with maple syrup urine disease is often known as *Menkes syndrome* and he described both the conditions. Incidentally, his grandfather conducted the autopsy on Ludwig van Beethoven.

Merkel disc
A form of nerve endings, sensitive to touch.

Mesulam's bisection test
This test is utilized to diagnose hemineglect in a subject. The patient is instructed to place a mark through the center of a line with a pencil. A displacement of the mark is observed toward

the side of the cerebral lesion in hemineglect, whereas in hemianopia, the subject turns his head and finds out the center of the line and places the mark precisely at the center, since he is aware of the fact that he cannot see in one-half of the visual field.

Mesulam's letter cancellation test A test for executive function where in a medley of letters, capital or small, the subject is asked to cancel with a pencil, a certain letter.

Meyer's loop The lowermost fibers of the optic radiation which pass through the temporal lobe and loop around the tip of the temporal lobe on their way to the calcarine cortex. They carry impulses from the inferior nasal quadrant of the retina and any lesion in the loop will result in superior quadrantanopia.

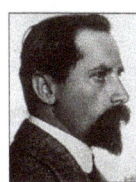

Adolf Meyer
(1866–1950, Switzerland)

Meynert decussation Decussation of the dorsal tegmental tract.

Meynert fasciculus A small bundle of nerve fibers passing from the habenula of the thalamus to the interpeduncular region.

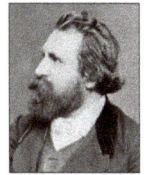

Theodor Hermann Meynert
(1833–1892, Germany)

Millard–Gubler syndrome A variety of crossed hemiparesis where there is ipsilateral 6th and 7th cranial nerve palsy and contralateral hemiparesis. The condition is usually due to a vascular lesion in the pons.

Miller Fisher syndrome The triad of ataxia, areflexia and ophthalmoplegia. It is considered a variant of acute inflammatory demyelinating polyradiculoneuropathy. It has been proposed that mismatch between proprioceptive sensation from muscle spindles and kinesthetic information from joints is the mechanism for ataxia, though others have observed MRI changes in the cerebellum. Anti-GQ1b IgG antibody in serum is positive in this condition and these are antibodies against ganglioside complexes. This is associated with the development of ophthalmoplegia.

Miller Fisher test The spinal tap test in normal pressure hydrocephalus to detect whether cerebrospinal fluid shunt operation will be effective. About 30 mL of CSF is obtained by lumbar puncture for three consecutive days and if there is improvement in the patient's clinical condition, shunt operation may be undertaken.

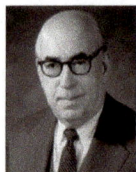

Charles Miller Fisher (1913–2012, United States of America)

Miller Fisher's One and a half syndrome In this condition there is no horizontal movement in one eye, while in the other eye only abduction is possible which shows nystagmus. In other words, there is conjugate horizontal gaze palsy in one direction and internuclear ophthalmoplegia in the other eye. The lesion is usually due to pontine infarction or hemorrhage affecting the paramedian pontine reticular formation and the medial longitudinal fasciculus on the side of the abducting eye.

Mills' disease A variant of amyotrophic lateral sclerosis, where progressive ascending, unilateral paralysis with wasting and hyporeflexia are the prominent features. Much later, the disease may become bilateral.

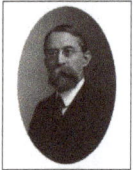

Charles Karsner Mills (1845–1931, United States of America)

Minkowski's rule Sometimes during recovery from cerebrovascular accident, neither the patient's mother tongue, nor the language most spoken at the time of stroke may recover first and thus, may not conform to *Ribot's law* or *Pitres' law*. On the contrary, psychosocial and psychosexual factors operate and decide an important role in the selection of the recovering patient's language.

Minor's sign In lumbosacral spondylosis, the patient may rise from the sitting posture by supporting herself on the unaffected side, bending forward and then placing one hand on the back at the affected side.

Miyoshi myopathy A variety of distal myopathy where there is wasting and weakness in the calf muscles. The patient is unable to stand on his toes. With time, it involves the more proximal muscles in the thighs and the buttocks. It is inherited as an autosomal recessive condition and the mutation is in the DYSF or ANO5S gene. It is a variety of dysferlinopathy (Fig. M.2).

Möbius syndrome A rare congenital disease with paralysis of the facial and abducent nerve.

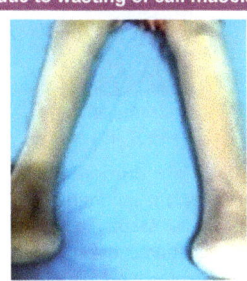

Figure M.2: Miyoshi myopathy. Note narrow long lower limbs due to wasting of calf muscles

Sometimes, 5th and 8th nerve are also affected. The children present with facial palsy and strabismus. Corneal erosion may result from inability to blink due to facial palsy. Pathologically, the 6th and the 7th cranial nerve nuclei are not properly developed.

Möbius-Poland syndrome This is the combination of the features of Möbius syndrome along with congenital absence or underdevelopment of the pectoralis muscle. Isolated underdevelopment of the pectoralis muscle is known as Poland syndrome.

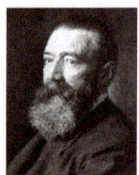

Paul Julius Möbius
(1853–1907, Germany)

Mollaret's meningitis Chronic or recurrent meningitis, often known as aseptic meningitis, the condition is diagnosed when pleocytosis is present in the CSF for more than 4 weeks. Headache, fever and neck stiffness are the common symptoms. Herpes simplex and varicella-zoster virus are commonly implicated as pathogens and acyclovir is used to treat the condition.

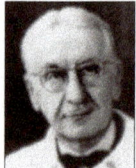

Pierre Mollaret
(1898–1987, France)

Monakow syndrome Contralateral hemiplegia, hemianesthesia, and hemianopia, following infarction of the anterior choroidal artery.

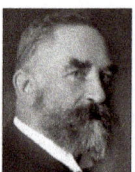

Constantin von Monakow
(1853–1930, Russia)

Monakow's bundle The other name for the rubrospinal fasciculus.

Monakow's fasciculus The other name for arcuate fasciculus which connects the Broca's area with the Wernicke's area. Lesion here leads to conduction aphasia.

Monakow's nucleus The other name for the lateral cuneate nucleus.

Moniz sign A variant of Babinski response where forceful plantar flexion of the foot may result in dorsiflexion of the toes in corticospinal tract lesion. It was described by Egas Moniz of Portugal and he introduced the practice of carotid angiography and prefrontal leucotomy in intractable schizophrenia, which earned him the Nobel prize in 1949.

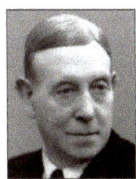

António Caetano de Abreu
Freire Egas Moniz
(1875–1955, Portugal)

Monro foramen The foramina which connect the lateral ventricles with the third ventricle.

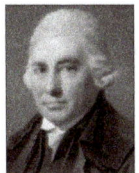

Alexander Monro
(1697–1767, United Kingdom)

Monro-Kellie doctrine Compensation for increase in volume in any component inside the cranium must take place by diminution in the volume of some structure inside, since the cranium is hard and inelastic.

Moro reflex A reflex in infants seen upto 6 months of life. A loud noise or passive movement of the head leads to abduction and extension of all four limbs. There is fanning of all the digits but the thumb is flexed. Usually, there is associated cry. Absence of this reflex indicates defect in central nervous system development, while its persistence after 6 months is also considered abnormal.

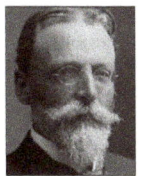

Ernst Moro
(1874–1951, Austria)

Morquio-Brailsford syndrome Also designated as mucopolysaccharoidosis IV, it is an autosomal recessive disorder in the category of lysosomal storage disease. The patients have large fingers like Marfan's syndrome, knock-knees, widely spaced teeth, flared ribs and cardiac enlargement. Atlantoaxial dislocation is a complication leading to quadriplegia. Like Hurler's syndrome, the cornea is hazy and the enamel of the teeth is thin. The joints are lax, hip dysplastic, and the feet are flat along with genu valgum. It is caused by malfunction of either galactosamine-6 sulfatase or beta-galactosidase enzyme.

Morton's neuroma Also known as Morton's metatarsalgia, it refers to a benign tumour of the plantar nerve, usually in the space between second and third metatarsal bones as a result of entrapment neuropathy by the transverse metatarsal ligament. It presents with pain and numbness. It is tested by placing the index finger and the thumb on the dorsal and plantar aspect of the affected metatarsal space and the forefoot is thereafter, compressed with the opposite hand by squeezing the metatarsal heads.

Morvan's disease Constellation of insomnia, neuromyotonia, spontaneous or stimulus sensitive myoclonus, hyperhidrosis, lacrimation, muscle cramps and delirium. It is an autoimmune or paraneoplastic condition and treated with plasmapheresis or immunoglobulin therapy. The term, Morvan's syndrome is also occasionally used to describe the insensitivity to pain in syringomyelia.

Mott's law It is the phenomenon of anticipation in genetic diseases, where the illness appears earlier in successive generations. Huntington's disease and spinocerebellar ataxia are good examples.

Müller's law Every nerve fiber subserves one modality of sensation, whatever stimulation its end organ receives.

Müller's muscle Also known as the superior tarsal muscle, it originates from the undersurface of levator palpebrae superioris and is inserted on the superior tarsal plate of the upper eyelid. It receives nerve supply from the postganglionic sympathetic fibers in the superior cervical ganglion and communicates with the oculomotor nerve in the cavernous sinus and end by supplying the superior tarsal muscle. It helps to keep the upper eyelid elevated and weakness of this muscle leads to partial ptosis in Horner's syndrome.

Müller's sign Early loss of abdominal reflex in multiple sclerosis.

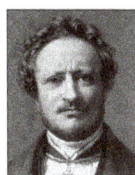

**Johannes Peter Müller
(1801–1858, Germany)**

Myerson's sign The other name for glabellar tap. Continuous blinking in response to tapping on the glabella as is seen in dementia or Parkinson's disease. This corresponds to the R2 component of the blink reflex.

SECTION N

Naffziger syndrome The other name for scalenus anticus syndrome, where there is spasm of cervical muscles following cervical spondylosis, cervical rib, etc. The spasm compresses the nerve trunks and nuchal and arm pain are the presenting symptoms.

Naffziger's sign Radiologically visible shift of the pineal gland as an indication of midline shift of the brain, like in subdural hematoma.

Naffziger's test Pressure on the jugular vein causes increase in intracranial pressure and leads to back pain in prolapsed intervertebral disc.

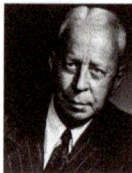

Howard Christian Naffziger (1884–1961, United States of America)

Negri bodies Eosinophilic cytoplasmic inclusion bodies in Purkinje cells in the cerebellum and the hippocampus in rabies. Negri himself initially thought these to be protozoal in nature.

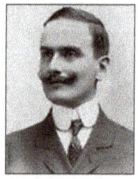

Adelchi Negri (1876–1912, Italy)

Negro sign The other name for cogwheel rigidity.

Neri's sign There are two such signs. One consists in spontaneous bending of the knee in the affected side in hemiplegia as the leg is passively lifted while the patient is lying down, and the other is in relation to lumbosacral radiculopathy, where forward bending of the trunk shall cause knee flexion on the affected side.

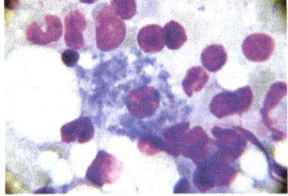

Figure N.1: Niemann–Pick disease, showing sea-blue histiocytes

Niemann–Pick disease (Fig. N.1) A group of inherited severe metabolic disorders in which sphingomyelin accumulates in the lysosomes inside cells. Hepatosplenomegaly and abdominal distension are common presenting features. Ataxia, dysarthria, dysphagia, dystonia and supranuclear gaze palsy are common neurological signs. Later, intellectual decline, seizures, early onset dementia develop. A curious feature rarely observed is the phenomenon of gelastic cataplexy, where laughter provokes sudden loss of muscle tone and fall. Genetically, it is an autosomal recessive disorder and mutation in the SMPD1 gene causes Niemann–Pick diseases types A and B, whereas, type C is caused by mutations in NPC1 and NPC2 genes. Histology reveals lipid-laden macrophages and sea-blue histiocytes in the bone marrow.

Nissl degeneration Degeneration of the cell body following damage to the axon, characterized by dispersion of the granular endoplasmic reticulum, swelling of the cell body and an eccentric nucleus in the cell.

Nissl granules Chromophilic granules in nerve cytoplasm which are composed of rough endoplasmic reticulum and are the sites for protein synthesis. They are absent in the axon hillock and undergo lysis in axonal degeneration. They are also known as tigroid bodies.

Nissl stain A stain devised by Franz Nissl, a histopathologist from Germany, meant for staining nucleic acid. The active ingredient is aniline, toluidine blue or cresyl violet. This basic dye binds to the negatively charged RNA or DNA in the nucleic acid.

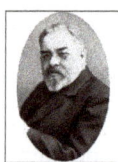

**Franz Nissl
(1860–1919, Germany)**

Nonaka myopathy A variety of distal myopathy, starting between 20 to 30 years with slowly progressive course, where the anterior compartment of leg is wasted. Consequently, dorsiflexion of the ankle is not possible. Other muscles in the upper and lower limbs are affected later but the quadriceps femoris is usually spared. Serum CPK level is usually within normal limits. Mutation is in the GNE gene and biosynthesis of sialic acid is jeopardized.

Nothnagel paralysis Paralysis of the oculomotor nerve and ipsilateral cerebellar ataxia or rubral tremor following lesion in the thalamo-perforating branch of the posterior cerebral artery.

SECTION O

Obersteiner sign A feeling that a stimulus applied on one side of the body is coming from the other side. This happens in tabes dorsalis and hysteria.

Ohtahara syndrome Also known as early infantile epileptic encephalopathy with burst-suppression, it is a variety of progressive epileptic encephalopathy. It presents within the first 3 months of life with tonic spasm, partial seizure, or myoclonic seizure and many of them ultimately progress to West's syndrome or Lennox–Gastaut syndrome. The EEG shows the typical burst-suppression pattern. There is severe atrophy of both the cerebral hemispheres and several genes have been identified. Anticonvulsants and corticosteroids are of limited value.

Ono's hand Selective flexion of the ring and little fingers in cervical radiculomyelopathy.

Onuf's nucleus Described by Bronislaw Onuf-Onufrowicz, a Russian neurologist, this is a group of neurons located in the lamina IX of the ventral part of the anterior horn cells in the anterolateral part of the sacral region of the spinal cord. Its function is the maintenance of sphincter integrity and the neurons contribute to the pudendal nerve. The cells are larger than the surrounding neurons and often designated as X cells. Located mainly in the S2 segment of the spinal cord they have larger Nissl granules. These neurons are spared in amyotrophic lateral sclerosis when motor neurons degenerate and the sphincters are spared even in the terminal stages. On the contrary, in Shy–Drager syndrome, characterized by sphincter incontinence, Onuf's nucleus is destroyed. Presence of urinary continence with consequent dry bed sheets, presence of sensation, and increased turnover of collagen fibres in the skin are the reasons why bedsores are usually not found even in terminal cases of motor neuron disease.

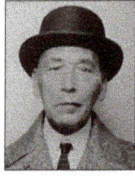

Bronislaw Onuf-Onufrowicz (1863–1928, Russia)

Opalski cell Large glial cells, derived from degenerated astrocytes with small, eccentric deeply staining nuclei in the periphery and granular cytoplasm found in basal ganglia, thalamus and the cortex in Wilson's disease and acquired hepatolenticular degeneration. It is believed that these cells block the entry of toxic substances into the brain.

Opalski syndrome When Wallenberg's syndrome is associated with ipsilateral hemiplegia, it is called so. The infarct spreads to involve the decussating corticospinal tracts at the lower end of the medulla of the opposite side.

Oppenheim's disease The other name for myotonia congenita.

Oppenheim's gait Wide swinging motion of the head, body, and extremities, often seen in multiple sclerosis.

Oppenheim's reflex Pressure over the anterior border of the tibia leads to dorsiflexion of the big toe in corticospinal tract disorder. Oppenheim observed the phenomenon in 1891, 5 years before Babinski described it but did not attach much importance to it since he felt that the sign was too inconsistent.

Oppenheim's syndrome Sclerosis of the spinal cord associated with tumor of the pituitary gland.

Oppenheim's useless hand Clumsiness of finger movements and manual dexterity following an attack of multiple sclerosis. This is sometimes associated with astereognosis. There is deafferentation and severe proprioceptive loss. This is due to deposit of plaques at the dorsal root entry zone and the posterior column in the cervical spinal cord.

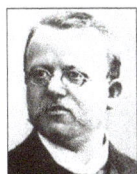

Hermann Oppenheim (1858–1919, Germany)

Oppenheim-Ziehen disease Dystonic condition described by Hermann Oppenheim from Germany in 1911. It is characterized by sustained muscular contractions leading to a bizarre posture. The movements distort the spine, limbs, hip and the gait may resemble that of a camel or *dromedary gait*. It usually begins in adolescence and the movements are relieved with sleep. It is inherited as an autosomal dominant trait and mutations are in the TOR1A gene, which is commonly known as DYT1 gene.

Orbeli phenomenon Stimulation of the nerve to a muscle together with its sympathetic supply results in increased contraction of fatigued muscles.

Orgogozo scale A scale devised for the assessment of impairment following cerebrovascular accident.

SECTION P

Pacchionnian granulations
The other name for arachnoid granulations, which are projections of the arachnoid villi into the dural sinuses helping in the drainage of cerebrospinal fluid into the venous system. They increase in number and size in old age.

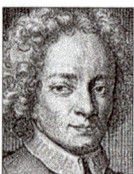

Antonio Pacchioni
(1665–1726, Italy)

Pacinian corpuscles (Fig. P.1) One of the four major mechanoreceptors in the mammalian skin. These are nerve endings which subserve vibration and pressure sense. These are oval shaped structures surrounded by a layer of connective tissue consisting of 20 to 60 concentric

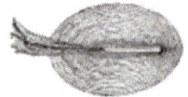

Figure P.1: Pacinian corpuscles, showing concentric lamellae

lamellae. During vibration these corpuscles respond by the opening of sodium channels which initiate the development of action potentials.

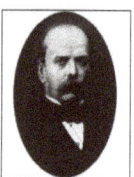

Filippo Pacini
(1812–1883, Italy)

Paget's disease Also known as osteitis deformans, it is an example of continuous excessive bone formation and destruction

Paget's disease

in the elderly, occurring simultaneously, and this may lead to the development of osteosarcoma in old age. The usual symptoms are bone pain, increase in size of the hat due to increase in the size of the head, fractures following osteoporosis, hearing loss due to entrapment of the vestibulocochlear nerve at the point of bony exit, visual loss due to compression of the optic nerves in the optic foramina and gross bony deformities. Associated complications are high-output cardiac failure due to hypermetabolic state, arthritis, renal stones as a complication of hypercalciuria, and spastic paraparesis following fracture of the vertebral column. Two genes in chromosome 5 and 6, SQSTM1 and RANK have been implicated in its causation, while others have postulated a slow viral etiology, like paramyxoviral or respiratory syncitial virus infection. The diagnosis is established by imaging, elevated alkaline phosphatase in blood and bone scan. Bisphosphonates, calcitonin, calcium and cholecalciferol are the drugs of choice.

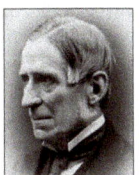

**James Paget
(1814–1899, United Kingdom)**

Panayiotopoulos syndrome

Also known as early onset occipital epilepsy, it is a variety of childhood epileptic syndrome which usually appears between 5 to 10 years of age. It usually starts as partial seizure and can thereafter spread to become generalized. More than half of the seizures occur during the first hour of sleep and profound autonomic symptoms, feeling of sickness and vomiting are common accompaniments. The EEG classically shows occipital spikes and centrotemporal spikes are sometimes seen. These discharges are often better seen when the child is not focusing on an object. The condition is not genetically determined and family history is mostly negative. Oxcarbazepine, carbamazepine, levetiracetam,

Paget's Disease

lacosamide and zonisamide are the preferred drugs. The prognosis is generally good (Figs. P.2 and P.3).

Pandy's test

Pandy's test A laboratory test to detect the presence of globulin, like in neurosyphilis, in the cerebrospinal fluid.

Figure P.2: Paget's disease. Note the enlarged head in the lateral view. The straight X-ray and the CT scan show thick skull along with erosions due to destruction

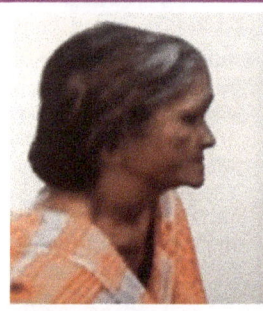
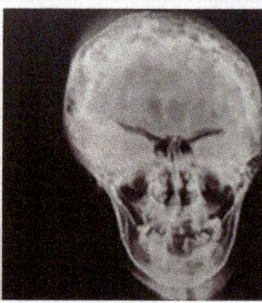

Figure P.3: Paget's disease

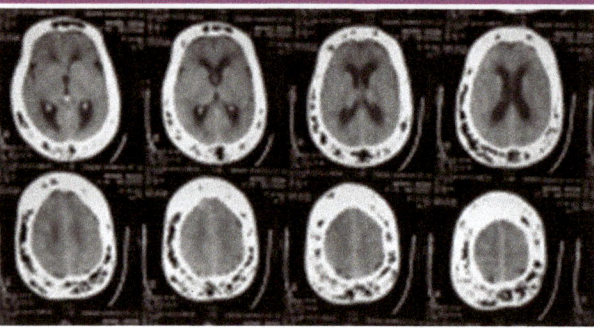

Papez circuit A neural circuit for the control of emotions consisting of hippocampal formation or subiculum and passing thereafter to fornix, mammillary bodies, mammillothalamic tract or tract of Vicq d' Azyr, anterior nucleus of the thalamus, cingulum, entorhinal cortex, and finally to hippocampal formation. Recent studies have shown that this circuit is more concerned with memory than emotions. Degenerative conditions like, Alzheimer's disease, Parkinson's disease, Korsakoff's psychosis, semantic dementia, transient global amnesia, etc. are often associated with degeneration of components of the circuit.

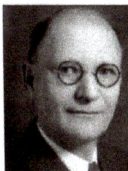

James Papez (1883–1958, United States of America)

Parinaud's syndrome Also known as the dorsal midbrain syndrome, there is inability to move the eye upward. Divergent squint, pseudo-Argyll Robertson pupil, and convergence retraction nystagmus are the other concomitant features. There is eyelid retraction, known as *Collier's sign*. The lesion is in the tectum of the mesencephalon, including the superior colliculus, oculomotor nucleus and Edinger–Westphal nucleus.

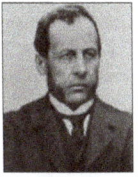

Henri Parinaud (1844–1905, France)

Parkinson's disease (please refer to any text book of neurology) There is no verified portrait of James Parkinson, even in the National Art Gallery. Photography was invented decades after his death by Henry Fox Talbot (1800–77) in England in the 1840s. Three photographs bearing his name can be traced by medical historians. The bearded man is in all likelihood, James Cumine Parkinson, a midshipman, who lost his interest

Parkinson's disease

in his vocation and later settled in the colonies of New Zealand and Tasmania. The one dressed in garish apparel with a cane stick in hand was a dentist who died in 1889. However, Simon RW Scott wrote that the elusive Parkinson is possibly represented in a painting in a book, The *Villager's Friend* and *Physician*, written and sketched by Parkinson himself, and he is seen lecturing before the gathering, though the evidence again, is scanty.

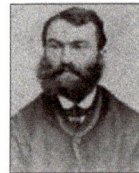

James Cumine Parkinson
(1832–1887, United Kingdom)

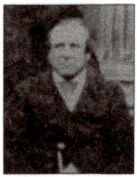

James Parkinson
(??–1895, United Kingdom)

Parsonage–Turner syndrome

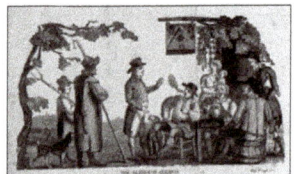

Village Physician
(1755–1824, United Kingdom)

Parry–Romberg syndrome A rare disease where there is progressive wasting of subcutaneous tissues, usually on one side of the face. An autoimmune mechanism is postulated and some consider it as a localized form of scleroderma. Sympathectomy can lead to this condition. The nervous system, eyes or the mouth may also be involved. Trigeminal neuralgia and migraine on the affected side are common associations. It is commoner in females and the usual age range is 5 to 15 years. Autosomal dominant inheritance is often observed. It is also known as hemifacial atrophy (Fig. P.4).

Parsonage–Turner syndrome The other name for neuralgic amyotrophy. Most of the cases are related to vaccination or recent infection and involves the brachial plexus. There

Figure P.4: Parry–Romberg syndrome. Note the hemiatrophy of the facial muscles as well as, thinning of hair in the left side

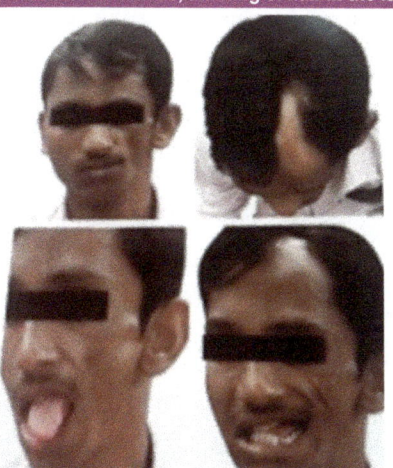

is history of severe arm pain, weakness and numbness. The affected muscles are atrophied and occasionally there is scapular winging. In more than 95% cases, the suprascapular nerve is involved and sometimes the subscapular and axillary nerves are also affected. Supraspinatus and infraspinatus are the muscles most commonly paralyzed.

Patrick's test A classic test to distinguish sacroiliitis from lumbosacral disc pathology. The leg is flexed and the thigh is abducted and externally rotated. The lateral malleolus is placed upon the knee joint and pressure is applied by the examiner over the knee. Pain is felt in sacroiliitis. It is also known by the acronym, FABER test (Flexion Abduction External Rotation) test.

Pavlov conditioning Also known as classical conditioning, it refers to the learning procedure toward a biological stimulus coupled with pairing with a neural stimulus. Ivan Pavlov's seminal experiment of ringing a bell leading to secretion of gastric juice in a dog, even when no food is offered attests the conditioning.

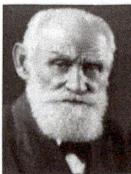

Ivan Petrovich Pavlov
(1849–1936, Russia)

Payne syndrome Involvement of the phrenic nerve, sympathetic chain, and recurrent laryngeal nerve in metastasis in the neck, usually from carcinoma of the breast. This results in diaphragmatic palsy, along with Horner's syndrome.

Pearson Marrow-pancreas syndrome A very rare mitochondrial disease of sideroblastic anemia, pancreatic dysfunction like, pancreatic fibrosis and type I diabetes mellitus, and neurological manifestations progressing to Kearns–Sayre syndrome.

Pelizaeus–Merzbacher disease A rare sex-linked disorder of the central nervous system where there is motor incoordination and delayed intellectual development. Head bobbing and nystagmus are the other features. MRI scan shows abnormal signal changes in the white matter. There is mutation in the PLP1 or GJA12 gene at the Xq22.2 region.

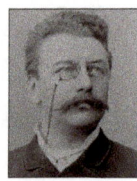

Friedrich Christoph Pelizaeus
(1851–1942, Germany)

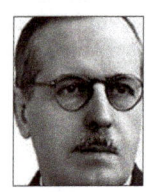

Ludwig Merzbacher
(1875–1942, Germany)

Penfield's motor homunculus

The map showing different anatomical area in the brain, subserving different functions. This was achieved by means of electrical stimulation in different parts of the brain.

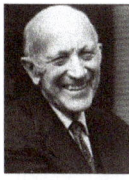

Wilder Penfield

Percheron artery

Percheron artery It is an anatomical variation where a single trunk arises from the posterior cerebral artery and supplies both thalamus and midbrain. It was described only in 1973. Infarction leads to vertical gaze palsy, memory disturbance and deep sleep from where the patient cannot be aroused easily which is collectively known as paramedian thalamic syndrome. MRI examination shows bilateral symmetrical hyperintensity, resembling a pair of spectacles (Fig. P.5).

Figure P.5: Percheron artery. Note the spectacle-like appearance in the thalami

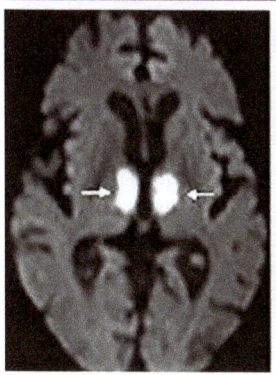
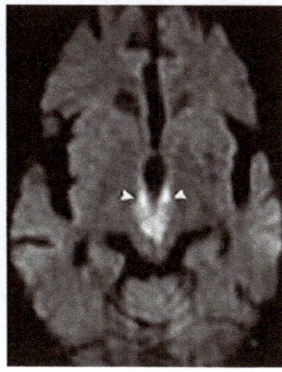

Neurology Defined

Perlia's nucleus A small group of cells in the somatic central column of the oculomotor nuclei. Since it is located between the two parts of *Warwick's oculomotor nerve complex*, supplying the two medial recti, it is supposed to be involved in ocular convergence and accommodation. The very existence of this nucleus has been debated in recent times.

Perry syndrome A variety of parkinsonism manifested as parkinsonian features, psychiatric changes like, depressive illness and apathy, weight loss and hypoventilation, often leading to respiratory failure. It results from mutations in the DCTN1 gene.

Phalen's test A sign of carpal tunnel syndrome where the patient is asked to outstretch the upper extremities and then flex the wrists as much as possible. This leads to tingling in the distribution of the median nerve.

Pick's disease Now designated as frontotemporal lobar dementia, it is variety of dementing illness where the frontal and the temporal lobes undergo marked degeneration. Unlike in Alzheimer's disease, where problems relating to memory are profound, this condition presents with language problem, emotional, personality and behavioral changes. Compulsive buying and gambling, impaired social conduct and disinhibition, inappropriate sexual escapades, vulgarity, overactivity and wandering are classical symptoms and there is often an increased liking for sweet edible items. Pick's disease presents as three distinct clinical syndromes like, frontotemporal dementia, progressive nonfluent aphasia and semantic dementia. An excess of β-amyloid protein is deposited in the brain and it is described as a taupathy with mutation in the MAPT tau gene. Classically, *Pick bodies*, which are intracytoplasmic argentophilic neuronal inclusion bodies, are deposited in the dentate gyrus of the cerebellum, hippocampal CA1 sector and the cortex. MRI scan shows gross atrophy of the frontal and the temporal lobe. Selective serotonin reuptake inhibitors are the treatment of choice (Fig. P.6).

Figure P.6: Pick's disease. Note the profound atrophy in the frontal and the temporal lobes and prominent Sylvian fissures

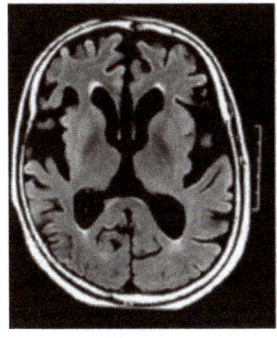
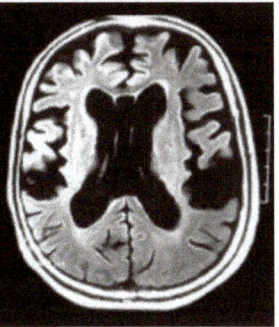

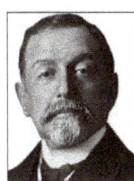

**Arnold Pick
(1851–1924, Czechoslovakia)**

Pick's pyramidal bundle Fasciculus pyramidalis aberrans.

Pitres' rule A dictum regarding the nature of recovery of speech in polyglots after an attack of aphasia. It states that the language which the affected person had been using most of the time before the attack, is the first one to come back.

Pitres' sign Lack of testicular sensation on squeezing in tabes dorsalis.

Pompe's disease Also known as glycogen storage disease type II, it is an autosomal recessive metabolic condition damaging the nerve cells and the muscles. There is an accumulation of glycogen in the lysosomes due to the deficiency of acid-alpha enzyme. The patient presents with the picture of myopathy and affects the heart, skeletal muscles and the nervous system. The infantile form is characterized by macroglossia, hypotonia, cardiomyopathy and failure to thrive, while in the late onset form cardiac involvement is not that common. The defective gene is located on the long arm of chromosome 17q25.2-q25.3.

Poser criteria A diagnostic criteria for multiple sclerosis devised by Charles Poser of Harvard in 1983 which replaced the much older and purely clinical, Schumacher's criteria. The team of investigators proposed that an attack is the occurrence of a symptom which lasts for more than 24 hours and clinical evidence is demonstrability of the signs and paraclinical evidence refers to the demonstration of a lesion by some investigations. Five separate subsets could be determined in the process like, clinically definite MS, laboratory supported definite MS, clinically probable MS, laboratory supported probable MS and no MS. This has, however, been supplanted later by the *McDonald's criteria* in 2003.

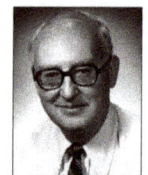

Charles Marcel Poser (1923–2010, United States of America)

Pott's disease Described by Percival Pott from St Bartholomew's hospital, London, it simply refers to tuberculous affection of the vertebral column. The lower thoracic and upper lumbar vertebrae are the ones most commonly affected. It occurs due to hematogenous spread of the tuberculosis bacilli which lodge in the intervertebral disc and spread to the lower half of the upper and the upper half of the lower vertebra, which along with the annulus fibrosus of the intervertebral disc, constituting one myotome having the same vascular supply. Collapse of the vertebral body leads to angulation of the spine, known as gibbus, and this presses upon the spinal cord, resulting in spastic paraparesis and sphincter disturbances from extradural compression.

Pott's paraplegia Paralysis of the lower part of the body and the extremities, due to pressure on the spinal cord from tuberculosis of the spine, or Pott's disease.

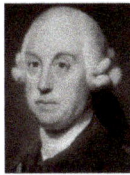

Percivall Pott
(1714–1788, United Kingdom)

Pourfour du Petit syndrome There is unilateral mydriasis, lid retraction and exophthalmos. Thus, it is the opposite of Horner's syndrome and therefore, it is often known as the *Inverse Horner's syndrome*. Thyroid carcinoma is often the underlying cause.

Prader–Willi syndrome A genetic disorder where there is obesity, type 2 diabetes mellitus, intellectual impairment and behavioral problems, characterized by voracious appetite. The forehead is narrow, hands and feet are small and the skin is light in color. Deletion in chromosome 15q11-13 from the paternal side is the underlying cause.

Pradhan sign A number of signs have been described by Sunil Pradhan from India. *Valley sign* refers to enlargement of the infraspinatus and deltoid muscles and when contracted they reveal partial wasting, leading to the appearance of a valley between two mounts, *Poly-Hill sign* indicates six bulges of the shoulder muscles and arm when the hands are abducted and externally rotated in facioscapulohumeral muscular dystrophy, *Calf head sign,* when an appearance resembling the animal's head is seen in Miyoshi myopathy on raising the arm with shoulders abducted and elbows flexed to 90 degrees, and *Diamond on quadriceps sign,* where a bulge resembling the precious stone appears on the anterolateral aspect of the quadriceps femoris on standing and slightly flexing the knee joints (Fig. P.7).

Figure P.7: Pradhan sign. Note the humps and the troughs in the shoulder girdle muscles, indicating selective atrophy and hypertrophy of the muscles, leading to the valley and polyhill sign. There is marked winging of the scapulae as well

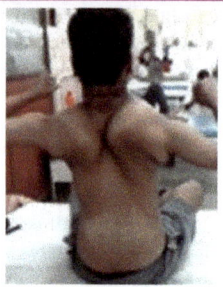

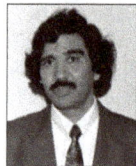

Sunil Pradhan
(1957–till date, India)

Pulfrich phenomenon A sign of optic neuritis in multiple sclerosis where, if a pendulum is swung in the frontal plane before the patient, the trajectory looks elliptical. It is a variety of stereoillusion.

Purkinje cells A group of GABA-ergic neurons in the cerebellum which are only the second largest cells in the human body after Betz cells in the motor cortex. Their dendrites arborize freely and have large number of dendritic spines. These are found in the Purkinje layer and each cell receives upto 500 climbing fibers and they send inhibitory influence to the deep cerebellar nuclei like vestigial, emboliform and dentate nuclei and they are the sole motor output cells from the cerebellar cortex. These cells are damaged by alcohol, lithium, autoimmune diseases affecting the cerebellum, spinocerebellar ataxias, multiple system atrophy, etc.

Purkinje effect Also known as *Purkinje shift*, it states that in the light adapted eye, the region of maximal brightness is in yellow color, while in dark adapted eye it is green.

Purkinje images Also known as *Purkinje–Sanson images*, are reflections of objects from the ocular structures. The first image is reflection from the outer surface of the cornea, the second one from the inner surface of the cornea, third one is from the anterior surface of the lens and the fourth one is from the posterior surface of the lens. All the images are true except the fourth one, which is inverted since it is concave outwards.

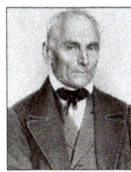

Jan Evangelista Purkyně
(1787–1869, Czechoslovakia)

Purkinje law of vertigo The direction of the apparent motion is determined by the position of the head during the rotation.

Purkinje layer The layer of large Purkinje cells between the molecular layer and the granular layers of the cerebellar cortex.

Purkinje's phenomenon A phenomenon of adaptation of the pupil of the eye to light intensity.

SECTION Q

Queckenstedt test A clinical test to diagnose block in the spinal canal inside the subarachnoid space. The patient lies in the lateral decubitus and is flexed to the intervertebral discs as much as possible, supported by an attendant. Lumbar puncture is carried out, the opening pressure observed, and thereafter, the internal jugular veins are compressed by an assistant. If there is no block, the cerebrospinal fluid pressure rises due to reduced absorption of the fluid through the arachnoid granulations and the manometric pressure goes up. In case of spinal block, this does not happen. It is worth remembering that positive Queckenstedt test is the normal phenomenon, as is positive Rinne's test. All other positive tests in clinical medicine represent abnormality.

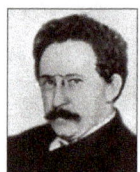

Hans Heinrich Georg Queckenstedt (1876–1918, Germany)

Quincke meningitis The other name for acute aseptic meningitis.

Quincke needle The classical lumbar puncture needle. Quincke performed lumbar puncture in the year 1891.

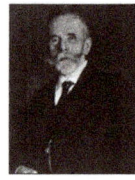

Heinrich Irenaeus Quincke (1842–1922, Germany)

Quinquad sign A sign in chronic alcoholism, where a crackling sound is felt when the examiner presses the open palm of the patient with both the hands.

SECTION R

Radovici sign The other name for palmomental reflex. Scratching the palm from above down across the thenar eminence causes ipsilateral contraction of the mentalis muscle, leading to puckering of the chin. This is a primitive reflex, found in dementia or pseudobulbar palsy.

Raeder's syndrome Also known as paratrigeminal syndrome, it refers to ptosis and meiosis as components of the Horner's syndrome, associated with unilateral headache localized to the eye. Sometimes, the trigeminal nerve is also involved. This is due to involvement of sympathetic nerve fibers in a lesion at the base of the skull.

Ramachandran sign A sign of right parietal damage where the subject is shown a mirror held to his right side and instructed to grasp a pen held towards the left side. On repeated attempts, he reaches for the mirror and neglects the pen on the left side.

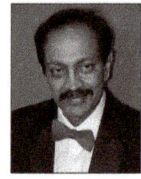

Vilayanur Subramanian Ramachandran (1951–till date, India)

Ramsay Hunt syndrome There are 3 entities in the name of James Ramsay Hunt. Type I is also known as dyssynergia cerebellaris myoclonica, described in 1921 and is characterized by myoclonic epilepsy, cerebellar ataxia, and action tremor. This is often the manifestation of Lafora body disease, dentatorubropallidoluysian atrophy, and celiac disease. Type II is the triad of involvement of the geniculate ganglion at the apex of the petrous temporal bone due to herpes zoster infection, facial paralysis, and vesicles on the pinna. Other features include hyperacusis, unilateral ageusia, decrease in tear and saliva production, and aural pain, while Type III is rare and is an occupational disorder where an artisan develops neuropathy of the deep palmar branch of the ulnar nerve. This is sometimes known as *Hunt's disease*.

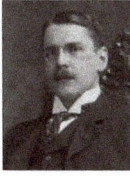

James Ramsay Hunt (1874–1937, United States of America)

Rankin Scale The modified Rankin Scale is used for measuring the degree of disability and dependence in daily activities after stroke or any other neurological catastrophe. It is graded from 0 to 6, (0) indicating no symptoms, (1) for ability to carry out usual activities despite some symptoms, (2) for slight disability, able to look after oneself but unable to carry out all activities, (3) for moderate disability requiring some help but able to walk without support, (4) for being unable to attend to bodily functions and needs, (5) for severe disability requiring constant care and attention, incontinent and bedridden, and (6) for death.

Ranvier node Areas of local constriction in the course of a peripheral nerve which lacks in the covering myelin sheath. In saltatory conduction, the impulse passes from one node to the other in order to transport of impulses along the nerve fibers.

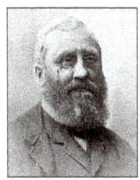

Louis-Antoine Ranvier (1835–1922, France)

Rappaport Disability Rating Scale A scale, as a kind of modification of Teasdale's

Glasgow Coma Scale, to assess continuous evaluation for prognosis of head injury. Special features assessed in the scale are toileting, grooming, feeding, level of functioning, and employability.

Rasmussen encephalitis Also known as chronic focal encephalitis, is an inflammatory condition characterized by frequent refractory seizures, motor regression, hemiparesis, encephalitis and dementia. The condition occurs in children and only one cerebral hemisphere is affected. It is divided into an acute stage, lasting for 4 to 8 months, when the inflammation is active with progressive worsening of the symptoms of hemiparesis, hemianopia, partial seizures, epilepsy partialis continua, and cognitive decline. Later, in the chronic stage, the inflammation turns quiescent and the sufferer is left with residual damage. Autoantibodies against glutamate receptor (GluR3) and NMDA receptor has been postulated. The condition is treated with steroids, intravenous immunoglobulin, and plasmapheresis.

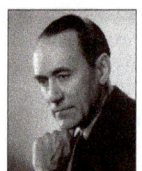

Theodore Rasmussen (1910–2002, United States of America)

Rathke's pouch An ectodermal evagination of the roof of the developing mouth which leads to the development of the anterior pituitary gland. Later, it is separated from the original site. Craniopharyngioma develops from the remnants of the cells in the epithelium in a cleft, known as *Rathke's cleft*.

Raymond syndrome Unilateral lesion of the ventral medial pons affecting ipsilateral abducens nerve fibres, and contralateral corticospinal tract, sparing the facial nerve. This is a variety of crossed hemiplegia.

Raymond-Céstan syndrome The condition where there is paralysis of conjugate gaze, ipsilateral abducens nerve palsy, and facial anesthesia along with contralateral hemiparesis. This is due to a lesion in the cerebral peduncles, involving the red nucleus.

Raymond-Céstan-Chenais syndrome Combination of cerebellar ataxia, coarse tremor, contralateral loss of all modalities of sensation, due to involvement of spinothalamic tract and medial lemniscus, contralateral motor paralysis, and paralysis of conjugate deviation towards the side of lesion due to involvement of paramedian pontine reticular formation.

Refsum syndrome An autosomal recessive disorder of phytanic acid metabolism where there is deficiency of phytanic acid oxidase enzyme with resultant accumulation of phytanic acid in the body. The onset is in childhood, course progressive and the presentation is usually with cerebellar ataxia, peripheral neuropathy, sensorineural deafness, and nystagmus. A striking feature is the presence of ichthyosis. Like Zellweger syndrome, it is considered as a peroxisomal disorder and the mutation is in the PEX7 gene. Treatment consists in advising diet free from phytanic acid and the patients are advised not to consume animal fat, tuna, cod and haddock.

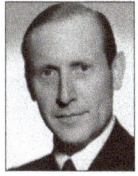

Sigvald Bernhard Refsum (1907–1991, Norway)

Remak sign Double sensation felt when a single sensory input is provided. It is observed in tabes dorsalis.

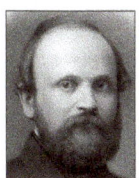

Robert Remak (1815–1865, Poland)

Remak's band The axis cylinder of a neuron.

Rendu-Osler-Weber syndrome Also known as hereditary hemorrhagic telangiectasia, it is an autosomal dominant neurocutaneous disorder with abnormal vessel formation in the skin, mucous membrane and organs like lungs, liver and brain. The clinical presentation is usually in the form of hemorrhagic episodes like, epistaxis, bleeding from the lips, fingers or mouth, hematemesis, melena, hemorrhagic strokes, high output cardiac failure due to the presence of arteriovenous shunts, etc. Many of the subjects have concomitant intestinal polyps which may bleed. Five genetic linkages have been identified so far and the fundamental problem suggested is angiogenesis.

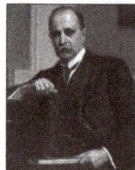

William Osler (1849–1919, United States of America)

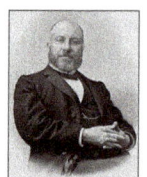

Henri Jules Louis Rendu (1844–1902, France)

Renshaw cell Interconnecting inhibitory internuncial cells connecting the dendrite entering the posterior horn of the spinal cord with the anterior horn cells. They receive an excitatory collateral from alpha motor neuron's axon as they emerge from the motor root and they send an inhibitory axon to relay with the cell body of the previous alpha neuron in the same motor pool. Renshaw cell inhibition thus represents a negative feedback mechanism and one Renshaw cell may be supplied by more than one alpha motor neuron collateral and it may synapse on multiple motor neurons. These cells utilize glycine as the inhibitory neurotransmitter. Strychnine acts on these neurons and block the action of glycine, leading to tetanic contraction and the toxin of Clostridium tetani acts in a similar way when owing to lack of glycinergic inhibition from the Renshaw cells, the alpha motor neurons tend to be hyperactive and they discharge continually leading to painful muscle contraction.

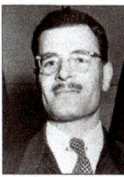

Birdsey Renshaw (1911–1948, United States of America)

Rett syndrome A neurogenetic condition, typically affecting the female sex. The disease manifests itself by 6 months of age and the course is divided into few stages. In Stage 1, the symptoms are mild and often overlooked. There may be subtle delay in development, limited eye contact, and reduced interest in handling objects. There is delay in growth rate of the head and constant ringing of the hands. In the Stage II which appears between 2 to 4 years of age, there is loss of hand skills and spoken language and characteristic stereotypy in the form of clapping, wringing, tapping of the hands. Apraxia, seizures, and autistic behavior appear in Stage III. In the final Stage IV, mobility is lost, the spine is curved, and muscular weakness, rigidity, spasticity, sleep problems, and abnormal posturing are the features. Stereotypic movements tend to decrease in intensity at this stage. The huge majority of the cases develop as mutation and the parents are usually genotypically normal. The genetic defect is in the MECP2 gene on the X chromosome in the long arm, which explains its sole occurrence in girls. Due to protean manifestations, the condition is now-a-days called *Rett Complex*.

Revilliod's sign Inability to voluntarily close the eyes on the paralyzed side in hemiplegia, while together the eyes close.

Rexed laminae There are 10 laminae or layers of grey matter in the spinal cord of which layer II is substantia gelatinosa, and layers III and IV is the lamina proprius. The intermediolateral column constitutes the lamina VII and lamina X is the neurons near the central canal.

Ribot's rule A dictum about polyglots concerning the recovery of speech and language following an attack of aphasia due to vascular insult. It states that the mother tongue is the first to recover.

Rich focus A tuberculous caseous granulomatous focus in the cortex or the meninges of the brain which may rupture into the subarachnoid space leading to tuberculous meningitis. This concept was in dissonance with the prevailing view that tuberculous meningitis was the result of vascular dissemination of tuberculous bacilli from pulmonary tuberculosis. As a matter of fact, Rich's focus appears as a consequence of hematogenous spread from the primary *Ghon's complex* in the lungs. This is one of the reasons that a subpial lesion which is more than 20 mm in size along with perilesional edema is diagnosed initially as tuberculoma rather than neurocysticercosis in imaging studies.

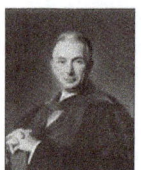

Arnold Rice Rich (1893–1967, United States of America)

Richardson syndrome A variant of progressive supranuclear palsy characterized by early onset postural instability, falls, vertical gaze palsy and cognitive dysfunctions, thus differing considerably from classical Parkinson's disease. Different clinical pictures of progressive supranuclear palsy have recently been described which differ from the classical description by Steele, Richardson, and Olszewski in 1963. Though they all have common histopathological, biochemical, and genetic features, the distribution of tau pathology is different. The classical form is now named *Richardson syndrome* whose incidence is lesser, while other variants are collectively known as PSP-P. The latter variety is characterized by asymmetrical onset, tremor, some initial response to levodopa and thus, often confused with Parkinson's disease. There is a male predilection for Richardson syndrome, while there is no such bias with PSP-P. Duration of the disease is also significantly shorter with Richardson syndrome. The mean four-repeat: three-repeat tau ratio is also different in the two conditions, being bigger in Richardson syndrome.

Riddoch phenomenon It is an ocular syndrome caused by lesions in the occipital lobe resulting in inability on the part of the subject in distinguishing objects. However, moving objects in the visual field are recognized, though their color is not identified. This is often seen in dementing conditions like posterior cortical atrophy.

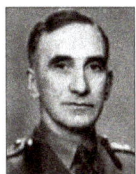

George Riddoch
(1888–1947, United Kingdom)

Riddoch's mass reflex In severe spinal cord injury stimulation below the level of lesion produces flexor response in the lower extremities, emptying of the bladder and bowels, and sweating of the skin.

Riley-Day syndrome Also known as familial dysautonomia or hereditary sensory and autonomic neuropathy, it is a disorder of the autonomic nervous system which hamper the development of the sensory, sympathetic, and parasympathetic neurons. There is congenital insensitivity to pain, hypolacrimation, episodic hypertension and postural hypotension, dysphagia, inappropriate thermal perception, ageusia, and gastroparesis. There is often delay in walking, unsteadiness of gait, and corneal abrasion. This is one condition where cervical and thoracic ganglia are atrophied and yet, there is paroxysmal hypertension. It is an autosomal recessive disorder caused by mutations in the IKBKAP gene on chromosome 9. Prenatal diagnosis is possible with amniocentesis and chorionic villi sampling.

Rinne's test A clinical test for the diagnosis of unilateral deafness, it consists in applying a vibrating tuning fork at 512 Hz frequency on the mastoid process and instructing the patient to indicate when he can no longer hear. Immediately, it is brought close to the pinna and if the patient can still hear, it indicates either normal hearing or sensorineural deafness. If it is absent, the patient is suffering from conductive deafness. It is based on the principal that air conduction is greater than bone conduction in the physiological condition.

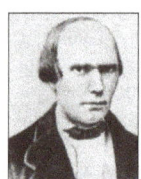

Heinrich Adolf Rinne
(1819–1868, Germany)

Rolandic area The other name for the motor cortex in front of the central sulcus.

Rolandic fissure The other name for central sulcus separating the motor from the sensory areas of the motor cortex.

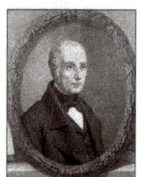

Luigi Rolando
(1773–1831, Italy)

Romberg's disease The other name for *Parry-Romberg disease*.

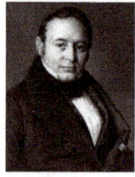

Moritz Heinrich Romberg
(1795–1873, Germany)

Romberg's test Also known as *Romberg's sign* or *Rombergism*, this is a classic test to assess the integrity of the posterior column of the spinal cord. The subject is asked to stand still with the feet together and the eyes closed and the physician stands behind, the hands kept close to the two sides of the body of the subject in order to prevent fall. The test is considered positive if the subject falls like a log of wood or sways considerably from side to side within 60 seconds. The physiological basis of the test is on the supposition that 5 components regulate normal posture and balance and damage to more than 2 structures is incompatible with normal stance. These structures are visual system, proprioception through the posterior column, cerebellar connections, vestibular system, and ligaments and muscles in the neck. If in conditions like, tabes dorsalis, the posterior column is wasted, other four components can compensate; however, if the eyes are also closed, the subject fails to maintain normal posture. The test can be rendered more difficult by asking the patient to stand with the toe of one foot touching the heel of the other foot, the so-called *sharpened Romberg's test* or asking him to stand on sponge or wool and thus rendering proprioception even more complicated in the *exaggerated Romberg's test*. If the subject is asked to stand with one foot directly in front of the other, arms folded in front of the chest and the eyes closed, a normal subject can withstand this posture for about 5 seconds. Failure to do so is a sign of sensory ataxia and is known as *tandem Romberg's test*. Wild swaying or gyrations without actual fall is sometimes referred to as *False Rombergism*, usually having some psychogenic component. It must be borne in mind that Romberg's test is a clinical test for posterior column dysfunction or sensory ataxia and not a test for cerebellar diseases. In the latter condition, the person sways even with eyes open and shall totter more if the eyes are closed. Thus it is positive in tabes dorsalis, Friedreich's ataxia, subacute combined degeneration of the spinal cord, etc. It was described by the German neurologist Moritz Romberg in the early 18th century and he was the first neurologist from Europe to write a text book on neurology.

Roo's test Also known as Elevated Arms Stress Test, it is a clinical sign of thoracic outlet syndrome. The patient flexes his arms and elbows to 90 degrees and the elbows are braced posteriorly. The subject then opens and closes his fists for 3 minutes. A positive test reproduces the patient's symptoms within 3 minutes.

Rosenbach's law In affections of the nerve trunk or nuclear center, paralysis of the flexor group of muscles appears later than that of the extensor group of muscles.

Rosenbach's reflex The other name for abdominal reflex. Rosenbach described it first in 1876.

Rosenbach's sign Fine tremor of the closed eyelids in hyperthyroidism.

Rosenthal fibers Cylindrical astrocytic processes, staining with eosinophilic dyes in fibrillary gliosis, found in *Alexander's disease*.

Ross syndrome A combination of Holmes-Adie syndrome, that is myotonic pupils and absent ankle or knee jerk, along with segmental anhidrosis, associated with compensatory unilateral hyperhidrosis (Fig. R.1).

Figure R.1: Ross syndrome. Note unilateral sweating in the right side of the back of the chest. Note dilated pupil in the right side as well

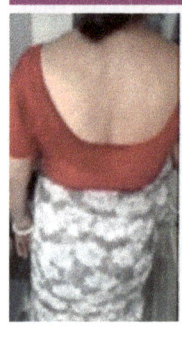
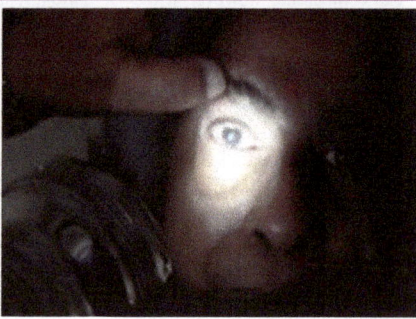

Rossolimo reflex A sign of corticospinal tract dysfunction where tapping the 2nd to 5th toes causes exaggerated flexion. This is one test for corticospinal tract damage where the great toe undergoes flexion and not extension.

Roth-Bernhardt disease The other uncommon name for meralgia paresthetica.

Roth-Bielschowsky syndrome A condition characterized by internuclear ophthalmoplegia with medial rectus paralysis for versions, intact convergence, and vestibular nystagmus in the abducted eye.

Roussy-Lévy syndrome A form of Charcot-Marie-Tooth disease, it is characterized by muscular weakness, sensory ataxia, areflexia, and pes cavus. Additionally, rhythmic shaking of the hands and gait ataxia are considered characteristic features. Nerve conduction studies show sensory nerve dysfunction. It is inherited as an autosomal dominant trait and duplication of the PMP22 or MPZ gene is implicated.

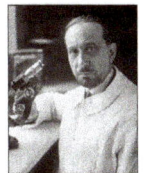

Gustave Roussy (1874–1948, France)

Ruffini's end organ Also known as *Ruffinian corpuscles*. These are cutaneous end organs sensitive to stretching of the skin and are most densely populated in and around the fingernails, responding to sustained pressure. They also act as thermoreceptors, responding to heat, though this view is no longer tenable and these are now supposed to be mechanoreceptors (Fig. R.2).

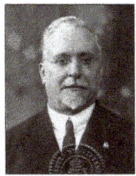

Angelo Ruffini (1864–1929, Italy)

Figure R.2: Ruffini's end organ

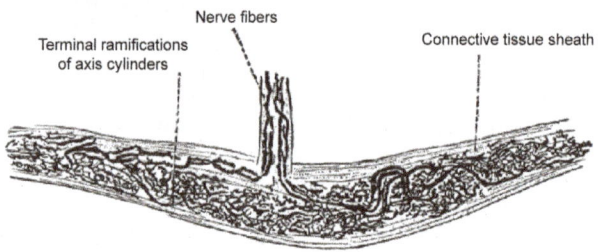

SECTION S

Sandhoff's disease A lysosomal lipid storage disease of genetic origin, clinically indistinguishable from Tay-Sach's disease. The enzymes beta-hexosaminidase A and B are deficient and these are required to degrade neuronal membrane component, ganglioside GM2. The progressive accumulation of GM2 leads to destruction of the cells in the central nervous system. The age of onset of the infantile form is at around 6 months with regression of milestones. The infants react sharply to noise, they are often deaf and blind, along with hepatosplenomegaly. Juvenile and adult forms are rarer, milder, and cognitive impairment, along with loss of muscle coordination are the predominant features. There are characteristic cherry red spots in the retina. The genetic lesion is mutation in chromosome 5 in the HEXB gene.

Sandifer's syndrome A condition where there is torsional dystonia involving opisthotonic posturing of the head, neck, trunk and the upper extremity, along with gastroesophageal reflux disease and hiatus hernia. The pathophysiology is not very clear.

Sanfilippo syndrome Also known as mucopolysaccharidosis III, it is an autosomal lysosomal storage disease. The age of onset is between 2 to 8 years with speech problems, hyperactivity and aggression, delayed developmental milestones and hirsutism. There are skeletal abnormalities, necrosis of femoral head, optic atrophy and deafness. The facial features are coarse with thick lips, and stiff joints. Hepatosplenomegaly is also common. There are 4 subtypes of this disease, each having different genetic inheritance in different genetic loci.

Sanger Brown's ataxia A variety of dominantly inherited spinocerebellar ataxia, it is characterized by ataxia, static tremor, brisk tendon reflexes, impaired posterior column function, and nystagmus. Often there are defects in the field of vision, absent pupillary reflexes, dementia, and sphincter disturbances in the later stages.

Santavouri disease Also known as muscle-eye-brain disease, this is a rare autosomal recessive congenital muscular dystrophy presenting with hypotonia, severe visual failure and uncontrolled eye movements with severe myopia. The mutation is in the POMGNT1 gene.

Satoyoshi disease A rare disorder of autoimmune etiology, characterized by diarrhea, painful muscle spasms, leading to dystonic posturing particularly in the thumb, alopecia, endocrine disturbances, amenorrhea, and skeletal abnormalities. The muscular spasms may number even upto 100 per day, each lasting for a few minutes, usually sparing the facial muscles. In the attack-free period, myoclonus may be a prominent feature. Antibodies to GABA producing enzyme, glutamate decarboxylase has been detected.

Scarpa's ganglion The other name for the ganglion on the vestibular nucleus in the internal auditory meatus.

Schaffer's reflex A sign of pyramidal tract dysfunction where squeezing the Achilles tendon elicits an extensor plantar reflex.

Schiff-Sherrington phenomenon When the spinal cord is severed in the mid-thoracic area or a little lower, the stretch reflex and postural reflexes of the upper limb are exaggerated, while if the transaction is at the sacral cord, similar features are observed in the lower limbs. These result due to release from the inhibitory influence normally exerted by the spinal segments below the transaction.

Schilder's disease Considered a borderline form of multiple sclerosis like, Balo's concentric sclerosis or Marburg multiple sclerosis, it is a rarer form of demyelinating disorder. Since the lesions are placed more occipitally, visual loss is a prominent feature and the other features are more or less like that of multiple sclerosis like, dementia, unstable gait, urinary incontinence and speech impairment, etc. The course of the disease can be monophasic, remitting and progressive. Corticosteroids, immunosuppressants and beta-interferons are the mainstay of management, apart from physiotherapy.

It is of interest to know that the condition adrenoleukodystrophy has some imprint of Schilder's disease as well. The disease described first in 1923 by Siemerling and Creutzfeldt was assigned an X-linked inheritance by Fanconi in 1923. A patient with encephalitis periaxialis diffusa, described by Schilder in 1913 was almost identical with what later came to be known as adrenoleukodystrophy and as a result sometimes the term 'Schilder's disease' has been assigned to this condition as well.

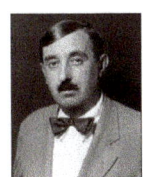

Paul Ferdinand Schilder
(1886–1940, Austria)

Schilder-Stengel syndrome A condition where the affected person, though capable of distinguishing the different types of pain stimuli, does not make any verbal, motor, or emotional response to painful irritation.

Schmörl's nodule Protrusions of the nucleus pulposus of the intervertebral disc into the vertebrae above and below and are identified in imaging as dense small structures. The nucleus pulposus is the embryological remnant of the notochord. These may often be confused with pathological lesions in the vertebral bodies. Schmörl's nodule may press upon the bone marrow leading to pain and inflammation (Fig. S.1).

Schneiderian first rank symptoms A bunch of symptoms in schizophrenia, described by Kurt Schneider, which includes auditory hallucinations, thought withdrawal, insertion and interruption, thought broadcasting, somatic hallucinations, delusional perception and feelings or actions experienced as made or influenced by external agents.

Figure S.1: Schmörl's nodule

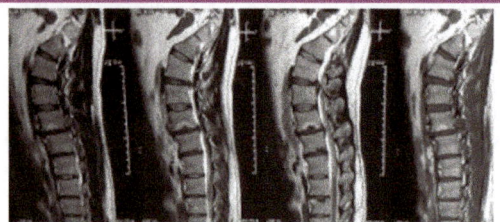

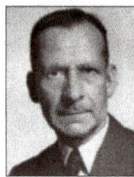

**Kurt Schneider
(1887–1967, Germany)**

Schumacher's criteria

The forerunner of the later developed *Poser's criteria* and the *McDonald's criteria*, this criteria was developed by George Schumacher. It is a clinical criteria which includes within its ambit, clinical signs of a problem in the central nervous system, dissemination in space characterized by clinical evidence of involvement in two or more areas, evidence of white matter involvement, dissemination in time, shown by either two or more relapses, each lasting for more than 24 hours and separated by at least 1 month, or progression of disability, age of the patient being between 15 to 50 years, and no better explanation for the illness. This criteria heavily influenced the later developed more precise and scientific Poser criteria in 1983 or McDonald criteria in 2001.

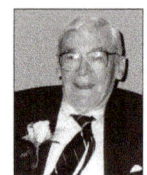

**George Schumacher
(1912–2008, United States of America)**

Schwabach's test A clinical test to distinguish between sensorineural and conductive deafness. A tuning fork is first placed over the mastoid process of the patient and then of the examiner. If the sound is heard for a longer time by the patient, conductive deafness is diagnosed. In the reverse situation, sensorineural deafness is the diagnosis.

Schwann cell Principal glial cells in the peripheral nervous system which lend support to the neurons. They wrap around the axons of motor and sensory neurons and produce the myelin sheath, often known as the Schwann sheath. They help in the saltatory, fast conduction of impulses across the peripheral nerves, and participate in nerve development and regeneration. They also provide nutritional support to the nerves, modulate neuromuscular synaptic activity and present antigens to T lymphocytes to produce cellular antibodies.

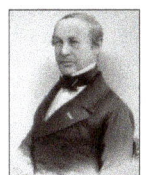

Theodor Schwann
(1810–1882, Germany)

Schwartz-Jampel syndrome Also known as chondrodystrophic myotonia, it is a rare genetic disorder whose main features are muscle stiffness, joint contractures, pectus carinatum, kyphosis, coxa valga, micrognathia, small and puckered face, blepharophimosis, and epicanthal folds. It is caused by mutation in the HSPG2 gene and inherited as an autosomal recessive disorder.

Segawa's disease A condition with onset in childhood where there is dystonia in the legs, typically occurring in one leg with diurnal variation, worse in the evening, accompanied by parkinsonian features. Some patients have hyperreflexia. It is an autosomal dominant condition with the genetic locus mapped to 14q21-22.2. It shows excellent response to small dosage of levodopa.

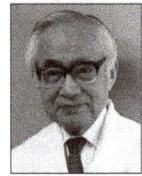

Masaya Segawa (1936–2014, Japan)

Seidel's scotoma A comma-shaped scotoma which is a superior or inferior extension of the blind spot, often seen in glaucoma.

Semon's law In the course of a gradually progressing organic lesion involving the recurrent laryngeal nerve three stages can be observed. In the first stage only the abductor fibers are damaged, the vocal folds approximate in the midline and adduction is still possible. In the second stage the additional contracture of adductors occur so that the vocal folds are immobilized in the median position. In the third stage the adductors become paralyzed and the vocal folds assume a cadaveric position.

Sheie's syndrome A less severe form of Hurler's syndrome where the affected individuals have corneal clouding and normal life span.

Sherrington's law of final common pathway All motor control signals ultimately synapse on α-motoneurons, which represent the final common pathway for the control of behavior by the central nervous system. Sherrington worked for the most of his time in Oxford, was the President of the Royal Society of London, and was the recipient of the Nobel Prize in 1932, along with Edgar Adrian. He coined the term synapse. He is universally regarded as the premier founder of neurophysiology.

Sherrington's law of reciprocal inhibition When a particular muscle contracts, the antagonist must relax to an equal extent, in order to facilitate the contraction smooth and purposeful. This is carried out by the mechanism of beta-innervation.

Sherrington's law of successive irradiation Strong voluntary contractions of a group of muscles will cause irradiation to other parts of the body leading to contraction of other muscles as well.

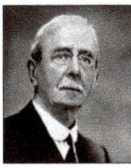

Charles Scott Sherrington (1857–1952, United Kingdom)

Shy-Drager syndrome A progressive disorder of the central and sympathetic nervous systems, described by Shy and Drager in 1960 in *The Lancet*. The symptoms include autonomic involvements like, dizziness, constipation, impotence, urinary incontinence, and later, speech, breathing, and swallowing difficulties along with anhidrosis. The affected subjects usually do not live beyond 7 to 10 years. Some patients present with parkinsonian features like, rigidity, bradykinesia, and cerebellar symptoms like, ataxia, and incoordination. When idiopathic orthostatic hypotension predominate the clinical features, it is often known as *Bradbury-Eggleston syndrome*. All these disparate presentations are now subsumed under one rubric of multiple system atrophy, where it is known as MSA-P, if parkinsonian features predominate, MSA-C, when the brunt of the disease falls on cerebellum and MSA-A, when the most distressing feature is autonomic failure, conforming to what Shy and Drager described initially.

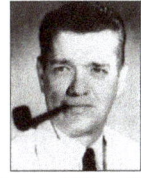

George Milton Shy (1919–1967, United States of America)

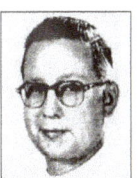

Glenn Albert Drager (1917–1967, United States of America)

Sicard's sign A modification of straight leg raising test where the great toe is passively dorsiflexed also.

Sjögren Larsson syndrome A condition characterized by leukoencephalopathy, delayed developmental milestones, spasticity in the lower limbs, seizures, ichthyosis, pruritus, erythema and scaly skin at the nape of the neck and the torso, which turns brownish. Ophthalmoscopy reveals tiny crystals in the retina. It is an autosomal recessive disorder with mutation in the ALDH3A2 gene.

Sneddon's syndrome A syndrome manifesting with stroke, transient neurological symptoms, livedo reticularis, or even larger livedo recemosa on the skin of the extremities. Other features are transient aphasia, cranial nerve palsies, headaches, and hypertension. The underlying pathology is a non-inflammatory arteriopathy. There is progressive thickening of the tunica interna leading to thrombotic changes and high dose warfarin is the therapy of choice.

Snellen chart A chart to assess the visual acuity. There are 11 lines of capital letters of progressively diminishing size, which is illuminated and kept at a distance of 6 meters from the patient and hung on the wall. The patient is instructed to read aloud the letters, known as optotypes, from above below and the ophthalmologist notices the level at which he starts having difficulty. The normal acuity is designated as 6/6, which means that a normal person has read a few letters correctly at a distance of 6 meters. But if one performs like 6/36, it simply means the concerned person read something at a distance of 6 meters which ought to have been recognized even at a distance of 36 meters, indicating poor eyesight.

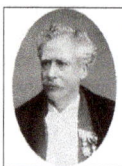

Herman Snellen (1834–1908, Poland)

Speed's test A test to diagnose bicipital tendinitis. The elbow is extended and supinated while the patient flexes the shoulder against resistance. This causes the biceps brachii muscle to move through the bicipital groove and caused pain in the arm anteriorly.

Spurling test Also known as cervical compression test, this maneuver is used to assess radicular pain. The patient's head is turned to the side where the patient complains of pain and extended, while the examiner applies pressure on the vertex. In spondylotic radiculopathy pain is reproduced in the corresponding dermatome.

St Vitus' dance The older and outdated name for Sydenham's chorea. Thomas Sydenham named the condition *Chorea Sancti Viti* in Latin in 1686, the first account of any movement disorder in the western world, and his account of the disease was also in the same language. An English translation is offered by Pechy in the celebrated textbook by Samuel Alexander Kinnier Wilson in his book published posthumously in 1940.

Steele-Richardson-Olszewski syndrome The other name for progressive supranuclear palsy described in 1963.

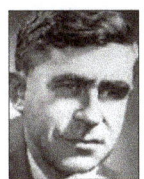

J Clifford Richardson (1849–1903, United States of America)

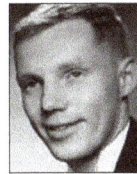

Jerzy Olszewski (1921–1981, United States of America)

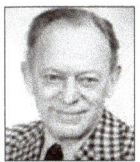

John C Steele (1934–till date, United States of America)

Steinert's disease The other name for dystrophia myotonica Fig. S.2.

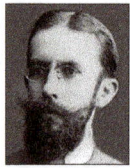

**Hans Gustav Steinert
(1875–1911, Germany)**

Strachan syndrome A nutritional deficiency condition first described in Jamaica, characterized by painful polyneuropathy, amblyopia, paresthesia, dizziness, glossitis, stomatitis, and sensory changes. Treatment consists in replacement therapy with components of vitamin B 12.

Stroop test A test employed to assess interference in the reaction time of a task. If the name of a color is printed in a different color like, the word red is printed in blue, and the subject is asked to name the color of the word, the time taken for the right answer is assessed. The chance of committing error is less if the color is to be identified in the same color as is shown. The hypothesis is that brain is capable of reading a word faster than it recognizes color and color recognition requires greater degree of attention. John Ridley Stroop of United States of America devised this test in 1929.

Strümpell-Westphal pseudosclerosis An outdated name for hepatolenticular degeneration by Adolf Strümpell and Carl Westphal from Germany. Kinnier Wilson severely criticized them in his seminal paper in *Brain* in 1912 and said that there was no evidence of hepatic cirrhosis in their patients.

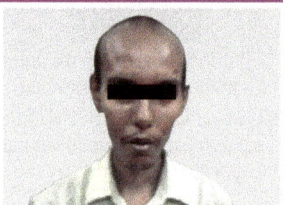

Figure S.2: Steinert's disease. Note frontal baldness, hatchet facies, atrophy of sternocleidomastoid muscles

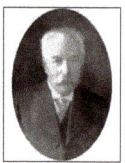

**Adolf Gustav Gottfried Strümpell
(1853–1925, Germany)**

Strümpell's upgoing toe phenomenon By pressing the anterior border of tibia the great toe moves upward, much like Oppenheim's reflex in pyramidal tract disorders. The Babinski's sign is known as '*Plantar response of Strümpell*' in the Netherlands for some obscure reasons.

Strümpell-Liechtenstern disease The other name for acute disseminated encephalomyelitis.

Strümpell-Lorrain syndrome The first description of the condition, hereditary spinal paraparesis.

Sturge-Weber syndrome Also known as encephalotrigeminal angiomatosis, this neurocutaneous syndrome is characterized by the presence of phakomatoses, port-wine stain in the face, glaucoma, mental retardation and leptomeningeal angioma of the same side. There are three types. Type 1 consists of facial and leptomeningeal angiomas, glaucoma and choroidal lesions, while type 2 presents with port wine stain and glaucoma is an inconsistent finding. Type 3 is characterized by extensive leptomeningeal lesions without any stigmata on the face. The facial stain is classically in the distribution of the ophthalmic division of the trigeminal nerve. Seizures and muscular weakness contralateral to the side of the port wine stain is characteristic. It is an embryonic developmental error in mesoderm and ectoderm and unlike other phakomatoses, it is not a hereditary disease and occurs only sporadically. Radiologically, there is calcification resulting from the leptomeningeal angiomas in the brain and are often known as *tram track calcification*, which occurs subcortically (Fig. S.3).

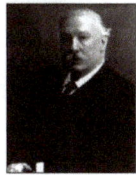

William Allen Sturge (1850–1919, United Kingdom)

Susac's syndrome A very rare form of microangiopathy characterized by encephalopathy, occlusion of branches of retinal artery and hearing loss with a female preponderance. The present idea is that antibodies are produced against endothelial cells in small arteries which leads to damage and the resultant symptoms. Slurred speech, headaches, migraine, hearing loss, visual problems are the usual presentation and they are usually self-limiting. Small vessel vasculopathy with arterial occlusion and microinfarction in the brain, cochlea and retina is the autopsy finding. The MRI scan feature is very characteristic and multiple punched out small hypodense lesions are seen in the corpus callosum. They often mimic the lesions in multiple sclerosis and acute disseminated encephalomyelitis but the lesions in Susac's syndrome are centrally located, while those in the demyelinating diseases, they often involve the undersurface.

Sydenham's chorea This is the first ever movement

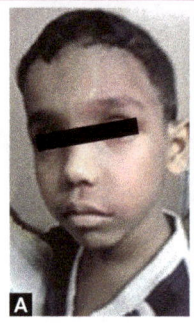 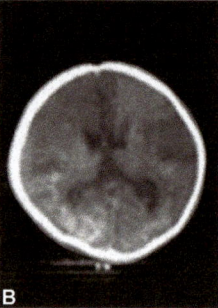

Figure S.3: Sturge-Weber syndrome. Note port wine stain on the left side of the face. CT scan shows extensive subcortical calcification

disorder described from Europe by Thomas Sydenham in 1686. It is a complication of childhood infection with Group A beta hemolytic *Streptococcus* and 20% subjects with acute rheumatic fever develop this condition. Sometimes, chorea can be only manifestation of rheumatic fever, known as *pure chorea*. The usual age of presentation is below 18 years and females are affected more. Apart from the involuntary movements some have dysarthria, gait disturbances, slowed cognition, hypotonia, and behavioral changes.

In recent times, one condition named Pediatric Autoimmune Neuropsychiatric Disorders Associated with Streptococcal Infections (PANDAS) has been brought to life, but it differs from Sydenham's chorea since motor problems are significantly absent here and tics or obsessive-compulsive disorders are commoner. The latent period from getting the infection and development of the neurological problems is less in this condition.

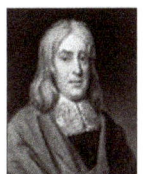

Thomas Sydenham (1624–1689, United Kingdom)

Sylvian aqueduct This duct connects the third ventricle in the diencephalon to the fourth ventricle in the medulla.

Sylvian fissure Also known as the lateral sulcus, this fissure separates the frontal and parietal lobes superiorly from the temporal lobe inferiorly. The insular cortex is located immediately deep to the fissure.

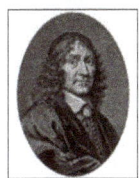

Franciscus Sylvius (1614–1672, Holland)

Symonds syndrome The other name for idiopathic intracranial hypertension.

SECTION T

Tangier disease An inherited condition which presents with peripheral neuropathy resembling syringomyelia with dissociated sensory loss and faciobrachial weakness, along with relapsing-remitting mononeuritis multiplex. Additionally, there is enlarged tonsils which are orange colored, hepatosplenomegaly, low serum cholesterol and raised triglyceride level.

Tapia syndrome A rare complication of airway intubation or cardiac surgery where there is extracranial involvement of the recurrent laryngeal nerve and the hypoglossal nerve. Clinically, it is manifested as vocal cord paralysis along with atrophy of the tongue.

Taylor hammer The first tendon hammer devised by James Madison Taylor of USA in 1888, where a triangular rubber is mounted on a small handle.

Tay–Sachs disease An autosomal recessive disorder of the nature of sphingolipidosis, characterized before the age of 6 months, seizures, deafness and problems in movement. The initial presentation is usually in the form of startle response to noise and other stimuli, listlessness and hypertonia. It is classified as infantile, juvenile and adult variety, based on neurological presentations. In the infantile variety, there is regression of milestones and death occurs very early. All patients have cherry-red spots in the macula of the retina. The pathophysiology is that excessive gangliosides are deposited in the surrounding retinal ganglion cells and this is the only area which is normal and the choroidal vasculature shows up in contrast to the surrounding pale retina. In the second variety, cognitive and motor deterioration with dysphagia, dysarthria, ataxia and spasticity are the usual features and death is by 15 years. The adult variety makes its appearance at around 30–40 years and the features are unsteadiness of gait, schizophreniform psychosis, with eventual wheelchair bound existence. The genetic locus is on 15q23 and the mutant gene is known as HEXA. There is reduced activity of the hexosaminidase A enzyme with reduced breaking of sphingolipids, which therefore, accumulate in the brain. This can be diagnosed by assay of the enzyme in fibroblasts or leukocytes.

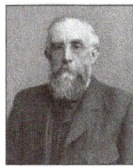

**Waren Tay
(1843–1927, United Kingdom)**

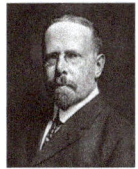

Bernard Sachs (1858–1944, United States of America)

Teasdale's Glasgow Coma Scale A scale for assessing the degree of coma, particularly following head injury that was devised by Graham Teasdale and Bryan Jennett from Glasgow in 1974. The parameters, eye movement, motor response and verbal response are assessed and the least value assigned is 1 and the highest value is 5. Thus considering the three items, the least total value is 3 and the highest one is 15. Subjects with values from 12 to 15 have 85% chance of survival, whereas those with values less than 3 do not usually have more than 5% chance.

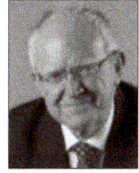

**Graham Teasdale
(1940–till date, United Kingdom)**

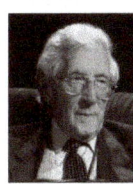

**Bryan Jennett
(1926–2008, United Kingdom)**

Terson's syndrome Vitreous hemorrhage in association with subarachnoid hemorrhage. It is caused by increased intracranial pressure as a complication of subhyaloid hemorrhage. Subhyaloid hemorrhage is supposed to be caused by infarction of the central retinal artery and its upper border is transverse in fundoscopy with the patient sitting. The other view is that blood in the subarachnoid space simply seeps down the space between the optic nerve and its covering sheath.

Thomsen's disease Autosomal dominant variety of myotonia congenita, where there is myotonia along with muscle hypertrophy, particularly in the thigh, calf and shoulder muscles due to continuous contraction of the muscles. Typically, the patients have difficulty in initial movement which improves with exercise and this phenomenon is known as *'warming up effect'*. The mutation is in the CLCN1 gene. The recessive variety of myotonia congenita is known as *Becker's variety*. The condition was first described by Julius Thomsen, a Danish German physician who himself suffered from the condition and it is estimated that 21 members of his family in a number of generations suffered from it (Fig. T.1).

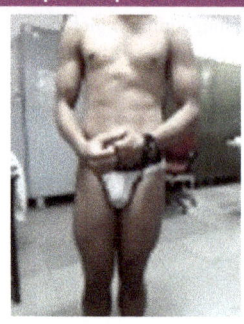

Figure T.1: Thomsen's disease. Note immense hypertrophy of the muscles, like a body builder. Note the extremely prominent quadriceps muscles

Tinel's sign Fundamentally, this detects the presence of irritated nerves but in general, this test is now known to diagnose irritative lesions in the median nerve. In essence, percussion across the median nerve over the carpal tunnel produces tingling sensation in the distribution of the median nerve in the palm.

Thus, in ulnar nerve compression in the Guyon's canal above the wrist the test can be positive.

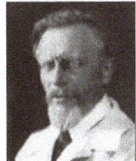

Jules Tinel
(1879–1952, France)

Tobey–Ayer test A clinical test to diagnose lateral sinus thrombosis. While performing lumbar puncture if pressure is applied over the internal jugular vein of the affected side, there is no increase in fluid pressure, while pressure on the normal side leads to increase in the pressure. Thus, in principle, this test is similar to *Queckenstedt test*.

Todd's paralysis It refers to focal weakness in a part of the body after an attack of focal motor seizure typically affecting one of the limbs. It usually subsides within 48 hours. It commonly takes place in 12–15% of cases. If the seizure is sensory in nature, originating from the post-central gyrus, sensory deficit can be the presentation, while aphasia is found in involvement of the conducting fibers. The commonest presentation is contralateral paralysis, though dystonic posture or clonic movements can occasionally be the feature. It is postulated that exhaustion of the motor cortex or increased inhibition is the cause of the paralysis. Others however, suggest that ischemia and reduced oxygen supply leads to this phenomenon. The condition was described by Robert Bentley Todd, London in his Lumleian lectures in 1849.

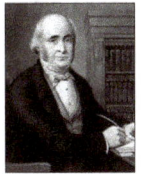

Robert Bentley Todd
(1809–1860, United Kingdom)

Tolosa–Hunt syndrome A condition characterized by pain in the eyes, increased on the application of pressure or on moving the eyes along with external ophthalmoplegia. The commonest presentation is unilateral headache, diplopia, vertigo or arthralgia. Usually, there is inflammation in the superior orbital fissure, or in the cavernous sinus and MRI scan of the orbit shows inflammatory changes. Non-steroidal analgesics, corticosteroids and azathioprine are the drugs of choice. The prognosis is usually favorable, though about 30% patients experience relapse.

Torkildsen shunt Ventriculocisternal shunt for the relief of the symptoms of hydrocephalus.

Tourette syndrome (the reader is referred to any standard textbook of neurology)

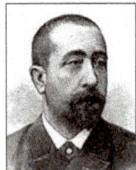

Georges Gilles de la Tourette (1857–1904, France)

Traquair's syndrome Also known as *anterior chiasmal syndrome*, this refers to compression over the optic chiasma leading to a classical defect in the visual field. The two optic nerves join to form the optic chiasma and thereafter, the nasal fibers cross to run in the opposite optic tract, while the temporal fibers travel in the ipsilateral optic tract, where it joins the nasal fibers from the opposite optic nerve. Thus the left half of the visual field ends in the right occipital lobe and vice-versa. The nasal fibers carry visual information from the temporal field and the temporal fibers from the nasal field. However, after crossing, the inferonasal fibers briefly enter the contralateral optic nerve looping back via the Wilbrand's knee, and then returns to the chiasma, though this view has been challenged in recent times. Therefore, a compressive lesion, usually a pituitary adenoma or craniopharyngioma compressing upon one optic nerve shall lead to ipsilateral optic atrophy, while compressing upon the Wilbrand's knee at the same time it will result in contralateral superotemporal scotoma, often known as junctional scotoma, a classical clinical syndrome.

Trolard vein Also known as superior anastomotic vein, it connects the superior sagittal sinu and the superficial cerebral vein of Sylvius.

Trömner's sign In pyramidal tract lesion flexing the fingers and then tapping the palmar aspect of the tip of the middle or index finger causes flexion of all the four fingers.

Trendelenburg's sign A sign in weakness of abductors of the hip, particularly gluteus medius and gluteus minimus. Gluteus medius helps to maintain the hip joint at the same level in the standing posture. This sign is considered positive if while standing on one leg, the pelvis on the opposite side of the stance, droops. The sign is found physiologically in pregnancy and in conditions like osteomalacia, rickets and in proximal muscle weakness of the lower limbs, like in Duchenne muscular dystrophy. This gait is often known as *Trendelenburg's gait* and the clinical examination, as *Trendelenburg's test*.

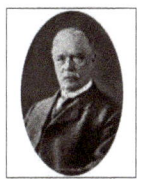

Friedrich Trendelenburg (1844–1924, Germany)

Trömner hammer A reflex hammer where there are two heads at the two ends, one being larger and the other smaller. The larger head is used to elicit tendon reflex, while the smaller one is used to elicit percussion myotonia (Fig. T.2).

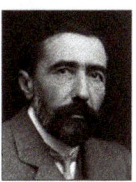

Ernst Trömner (1868–1930, Germany)

Trotter's syndrome A group of symptoms in advanced nasopharyngeal carcinoma like, unilateral conductive deafness due to middle ear effusion,

Figure T.2: Trömner hammer

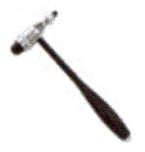

trigeminal neuralgia, paralysis of soft palate, difficulty in jaw opening, etc.

Tullio phenomenon This refers to vertigo, dizziness, nausea and nystagmus, induced by sound. It is usually caused by a fistula in the middle or inner ear often caused by barotrauma, fenestration surgery, syphilis, Lyme disease or superior semicircular canal dehiscence syndrome.

Turck's bundle The fibres from the corticospinal tract that do not cross at the lower medulla, but descend ipsilaterally to synapse in the same side. The decussation of the huge majority of the fibres in the medulla, which cross to the opposite side, is often known as *Mistichelli crossing*. Some residual fibres which descend ipsilaterally but cross towards the opposite side at the end to synapse with the anterior horn cells are known as the *anterolateral tract of Barnes*.

SECTION U

Udd myopathy A rare form of distal childhood muscular dystrophy characterized by weakness of dorsiflexion of ankle and inability to walk on heels, indicating weakness of the anterior compartment of the tibial group of muscles. There is foot drop and clumsiness during walking. It may remain unnoticed till later age. It is inherited as an autosomal dominant trait caused by mutations in the protein titin, on the long arm of chromosome 2q24.3.

Uhthoff's phenomenon Worsening of the neurological symptoms of multiple sclerosis on exposure to hot weather. They include, visual obscuration, fatigue, pain, urinary urgency, flexor spasms, etc. These symptoms disappear when the temperature is restored to normal. It is possibly due to the influence of temperature on nerve conduction. Since physical exercise raises body core temperature, caution must be exercised while advising physiotherapy for these patients. *Inverse Uhthoff sign* refers to the curious condition where paradoxically symptoms improve with increase in temperature.

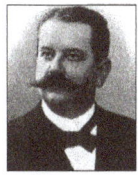

**Wilhelm Uhthoff
(1853–1927, Germany)**

Ullmann syndrome A congenital condition where there are multiple angiomatous malformations in the brain along with dural abnormalities. Probably it is a form of Rendu-Osler-Weber syndrome

Ullrich congenital myopathy The features include abnormal facial features, thin habitus with generalized muscular wasting, protuberant calcanei, predominantly distal weakness,

Ullrich congenital myopathy

contractures at shoulder, elbow, hip and knee, kyphoscoliosis and laxity of joints. This is inherited as an autosomal dominant gene and the chromosomal locus is at 21q22.3 and 2q37. The mutation is in COL6A1, COL6A2 and COL6A3 genes (Figs. U.1 and U.2).

> Figure U.1: Ullrich congenital myopathy. Note abnormal facial contour, contracture at the neck, kyphoscoliosis and generalized muscular wasting

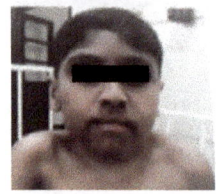

> Figure U.2: Ullrich congenital myopathy

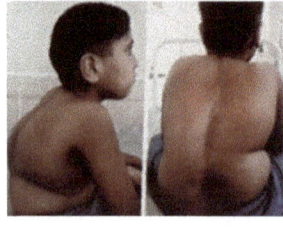

Uner Tan syndrome

An extremely rare disorder, first identified by the Turkish evolutionary biologist, Uner Tan in this century. Persons affected walk with a quadripedal gait, severe mental derangement and are afflicted with primitive speech. He considered it as an instance of *reverse evolution*. The affected subjects walk with their palm glued to the surface. Males are more affected. Other biologists argue that it is not a case of atavism, and on the contrary, they proposed that it is a problem of balance and therefore, gait. PET scan shows hypoperfusion in the cerebellum and in some areas of the cortex and MRI scan clearly shows profound cerebellar atrophy. Considered as an autosomal recessive disease, there is mutation in the TUBB2B gene which leads to damage to the cerebellum. G Wali from Belgaum has described such a case from India.

Unterberger's test

A clinical test to assess vertigo of peripheral origin. The patient is asked to close the eyes and walk straight with the hands outstretched in front. In labyrinthine disorder, the patient veers toward the ipsilateral side. PET scan has revealed hypoperfusion in the cerebellum and parts of the cerebrum and there is cerebral atrophy.

Usher syndrome Also known as *Hallgren syndrome*, it is a rare autosomal recessive condition caused by mutation in any one of at least 11 genes. There is progressive blindness from retinitis pigmentosa, sensorineural deafness, vestibular impairment, cerebellar ataxia and mental retardation. Four different types have been described depending upon the clinical features and genetic nature.

SECTION V

Valsalva maneuver Forcible expiration through a closed glottis leading to rise in intrathoracic pressure. In a normal subject it results in a rise in the pressure and a transient rise in blood pressure, known as *phase I*. Thereafter, there is reduction in venous return to the heart and that leads to an increase in the pulse rate (*phase II*). As the pressure is released, there is further increase in pulse rate and decrease in blood pressure (*phase III*), followed by return of blood pressure to the normal level after an initial overshoot, represented graphically by a transient spike, while the pulse rate falls. Abnormalities in these changes suggests parasympathetic nervous system disturbance.

Van Bogaert encephalitis The other name for subacute sclerosing encephalitis.

Van der Knapp disease A variety of megalencephalic leukoencephalopathy with subcortical cysts, found classically in the temporal lobe along with symmetrical white matter edema. It is a rare autosomal recessive disorder, characterized by macrocephaly that either presents at birth or develops during infancy. In India it has been described in the Agarwal community in India by Singhal et al. from Mumbai and one case has been reported in a Bengali girl by Bhattacharyya. This disease typically presents with a history of delayed motor milestones in affected children (Fig. V.1).

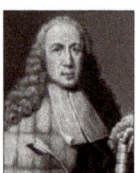

Antonia Mario Valsalva
(1666–1723, Italy)

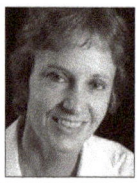

Van der Knapp
(1958–till date, Holland)

Figure V.1: Van der Knapp disease. Note the enlarged head in the lateral view. The MRI shows anterior white matter edema and bilateral temporal cysts in the cerebral cortex

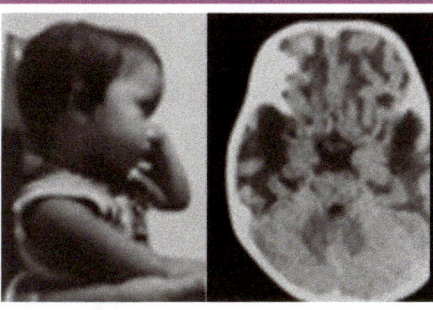

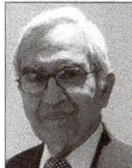

**Bhim Singhal
(1933–till date, India)**

Vernet syndrome A jugular foraminal syndrome characterized by paralysis of 9th, 10th and 11th nerve, with or without the 12th nerve.

Vical's syndrome In primary hyperparathyroidism, there may be weakness, muscular atrophy and fasciculations, thus resembling motor neuron disease.

Vicq d'Azyr tract The other name for mammillothalamic Tract.

Villaret syndrome Also known as retroparotid space syndrome, it is characterized by unilateral paralysis of 9th, 10th, 11th, and 12th cranial nerves along with Horner's syndrome. Facial nerve involvement is an occasional feature.

Virchow–Robin space An immunological space in the brain between an artery, a vein, and pia mater. As the arteries pierce deep into the substance of the brain, they carry a sheath of pia mater along with them. The perivascular space created thereby is the perivascular cuff which is the locus for leucocytes to aggregate in infective conditions. One function of Virchow–Robin space is in the regulation of fluid movement in the nervous system and its drainage into the cervical lymph nodes. Phagocytosis of cell debris by leukocytes and immunoregulation are other important functions. These spaces are visible as round structures in MRI.

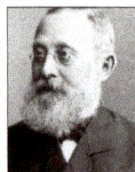

Rudolf Virchow
(1821–1902, Germany)

Vogt syndrome Also known as Vogt-Wilson syndrome, this is manifested as cerebral palsy, athetosis, chorea, dystonia, and accompanied by mental retardation. Pathologically, there are myelinated fibers inside the corpus striatum.

Vogt–Koyanagi–Harada syndrome This is a multi-system disorder, presumably of autoimmune origin, which affects the pigmented tissues. There is bilateral uveitis with blurring of vision, tinnitus, vertigo, hyperacusis, meningitis, cranial nerve palsy and cutaneous features like, vitiligo, alopecia and poliosis. Cerebrospinal fluid shows pleocytosis.

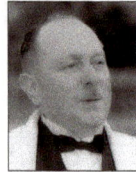

Alfred Vogt
(1879–1943, Germany)

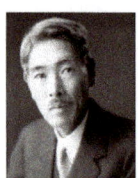

Yoshizo Koyanagi
(1880–1954, Japan)

Von Economo's disease

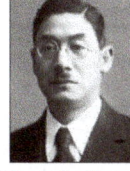

Einosuke Harada
(1892–1946, Japan)

Von Economo's disease Also known as encephalitis lethargica this condition was described by the Romanian neuropathologist Constantin von Economo in 1917. An epidemic of encephalitis swept the entire world between 1915 and 1926 and nearly 5 million people were affected. Those who survived developed postencephalitic Parkinsonism in the early 1930s. The precise etiology is unknown but an autoimmune response to viral and bacterial infections has been postulated. The link between influenza virus and the disease is established and post-encephalitic parkinsonism following the epidemic of influenza, and encephalitis lethargica clearly attests the hypothesis. Enterococcus and Diplococcus have also been incriminated in the aetiopathogenesis in recent times. Von Economo collected and analyzed thousands of cases and classified them into three clinical syndromes, namely, somnolent-opthalmoplegic, hyperkinetic and amyostatic forms.

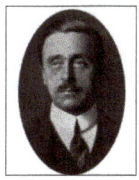

Constantin von Economo
(1876–1931, Austria)

Von Eulenburg's disease

Von Eulenburg's disease Also known as paramyotonia congenita it is a rare autosomal dominant condition, caused by mutation in the sodium-channel gene SCN4A, and characterized by muscle cramps or myotonia. The myotonia seems paradoxical in the sense that whereas other myotonias improve with exercise, it worsens in this condition. It can also be induced by exposure to cold weather. It has been reported that consumption of carrots and watermelon can lead to the condition. Typically, the patients complain of muscle stiffness and focal weakness. Acetazolamide and mexiletine can be used with limited success.

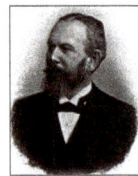

Albert von Eulenburg
(1840–1917, Germany)

Von Hippel–Lindau disease

Also known as cerebello-retinal hemangiomatosis, this is a neurocutaneous syndrome or phakomatoses inherited in an autosomal dominant nature with the chromosomal locus at 3p25.3. The clinical features include, angiomatosis, hemangioblastomas, pheochromocytoma, renal cell carcinoma, pancreatic cysts, and papillary cystadenoma of the epididymis. Most of the patients present with only one variety of tumor only.

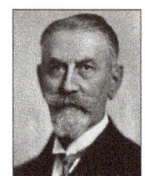

Eugen von Hippel
(1867–1939, Germany)

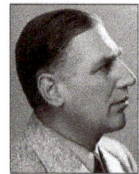

Arvid Vilhelm Lindau
(1892–1958, Sweden)

Von Recklinghausen's disease

Also known as neurofibromatosis type 1 (NF-1), it is an autosomal dominant disorder having multisystem expression. Congenital musculoskeletal disorders, cutaneous café au-lait spots, and multiple tumors arising from the peripheral nerves, retinal tumors, Lisch nodules on the iris, axillary freckles, known as *Crowe's sign*, learning disabilities, malignant transformation into neurofibrosarcoma, are the common presentations. Kyphoscoliosis, bare orbit due to agenesis of sphenoidal wing are the common skeletal abnormalities, while optic nerve glioma is an accompaniment. The café-au-lait spots are more than 1.5 cm in size, increase in size during pregnancy, and should be more than 6 at the back in one side. The mutation is on chromosome 17 and the mutant gene produces an abnormal protein, neurofibromin, needed for the normal functions in many human cells. The condition should not be confused with von Recklinghausen's disease of the bone or osteitis fibrosa cystica, where there are cystic cavities in the bones as a complication of hyperparathyroidism (Fig. V.2).

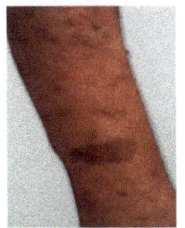

Figure V.2: Von Recklinghausen's disease

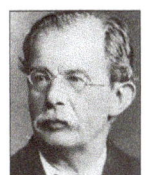

Friedrich Daniel von Recklinghausen (1833–1910, Germany)

Vulpian sign Conjugate deviation of eyes towards the side of acute cerebral lesion.

Vulpian-Bernhardt syndrome Variant of motor neuron disease characterized by involvement of the shoulder girdle and upper limbs without much involvement of the lower limbs or bulbar muscles (Fig. V.3).

Vulpian–Heidenhain–Sherrington phenomenon Slow contraction of denervated skeletal muscle by stimulating autonomic cholinergic fibers innervating its blood vessels.

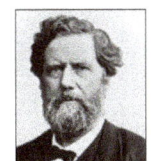

Edmé Félix Alfred Vulpian (1826–1887, France)

Figure V.3: Vulpian-Bernhardt syndrome. Note gross muscular wasting in the proximal muscles of the shoulder girdles, trunk, and shoulder muscles. Electromyography proved it to be a case of chronic anterior horn cell degeneration

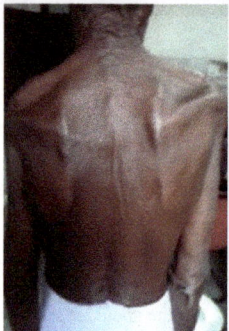
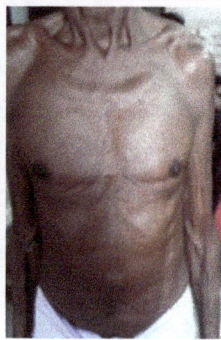

SECTION W

Wada test A test to ascertain cerebral dominance in terms of language and memory representation in the cerebral hemispheres. It is also known as the *sodium amytal test*. Sodium amobarbital is injected into one internal carotid artery and the procedure blocks the functions of that hemisphere which it supplies. The physician looks when is the speech affected and that localizes the speech area. The test is also applied before epilepsy surgery to locate the locus of discharge. It is fraught with the danger of drastic personality changes and disinhibition syndrome. Return of speech faculty is also a concomitant problem.

Wadia's variant of spinocerebellar ataxia A variety of spinocerebellar ataxia, described in India by NH Wadia in 1971 in *Brain*, characterized by slow horizontal saccades along with head jerk and an obligatory blink, when asked to fixate the gaze on a distant object. So slow and uniform is the movement of the eye that he described it *'as if floating in oil'*. Peripheral neuropathy is a common accompaniment, as are other cerebellar signs. It has been later shown to be a variety of spinocerebellar ataxia type 2 and the chromosomal locus is in chromosome 12. However, later works indicated that such slow saccades are also seen in other varieties of spinocerebellar ataxias like, SCA1 and SCA3. Further works have shown ethnic variations in the genetic patterns in India. Ranganath from Tamil Nadu showed that SCA1 is the commonest variety in Tamil Brahmins, while Chakraborty et al, and Bhattacharyya et al, from Kolkata found in independent studies that SCA 3 outnumbers the other varieties in ethnic Bengalees.

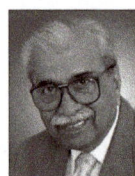

Noshir Hormusjee Wadia
(1925–2016, India)

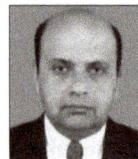

Ambar Chakravarty
(1948–Till Date, India)

Wagner-Jauregg treatment It refers to pyrotherapy as a measure for treating general paralysis of the insane. In 1917, Wagner-Jauregg from Austria demonstrated the therapeutic effect of inoculation of the malaria parasite, *Plasmodium vivax*, by inducing fever in neurosyphilis, and malaria was later treated with quinine, though initially he tested the patients with tuberculin and erysipelas which turned out to be abortive. This work fetched him the Nobel Prize in 1927. The procedure however, was fraught with the risk of death in about 15% of subjects and hence, it is no longer in use.

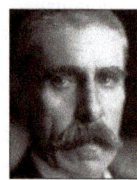

Julius Wagner-Jauregg
(1857–1940, Austria)

Walker–Warburg disease An inherited autosomal recessive variety of congenital muscular dystrophy characterized by muscle wasting, hypotonia, lissencephaly, hydrocephalus, seizures, microphthalmia, buphthalmos, cataracts and coloboma of the optic nerves. The mutations are in the POMT1, POMT2, ISPD, FKTN and LARGE1 gene.

Wallenberg's syndrome Also known as *lateral medullary syndrome*, it is a condition caused due to ischemic damage to the lateral part of the medulla oblongata, due to blockage in the posterior inferior cerebellar artery in most of the cases, or the vertebral artery. There is sensory loss in the trunk and extremities in the contralateral side owing to involvement of the spinothalamic tract, while facial sensory deficit is in the ipsilateral side due to the involvement of the spinal tract of trigeminal nerve, or the quintothalamic tract. Other features are dysphagia, staccato speech, ataxia, vertigo, nystagmus due to involvement of cerebellar fibers, Horner's syndrome due to involvement of the sympathetic trunk, intractable hiccough, and inability to sneeze due to paralysis of the vagus nerve.

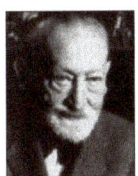

Adolf Wallenberg
(1862–1949, Germany)

Wallerian degeneration

Degenerative process which occurs with the distal portion of axon when a nerve fiber is injured. Thus, it occurs further from the cell body of the neuron. The condition is also known as orthograde or anterograde degeneration. When axonal transport is impaired the condition is known as *Wallerian-like degeneration*. It usually begins 24–36 hours of the trauma and before the degeneration starts the distal stump is electrically excitable. Thereafter, the axonal skeleton disintegrates and axonal membrane breaks down. This is followed by degradation of the myelin sheath which is infiltrated with inflammatory cells and macrophages. The Schwann cells also help to clear the remaining debris and help in the production of myelin sheath, which align in tubes, known as *Bünger's bands*, and within 4 days of the injury, the portion of the nerve proximal to the lesion sends out sprouting growths at the rate of 1 mm per day, toward the tubes. They are further attracted by growth factors produced by the Schwann cells and finally reach the target organ.

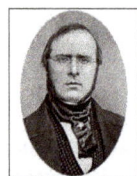

Augustus Volney Waller (1816–1870, United Kingdom)

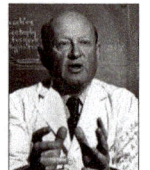

Robert Wartenberg (1887–1956, United States of America)

Wartenberg pendulum test
A clinical test to distinguish between the increase in muscle tone in upper motor neuron disorders and between spasticity from pyramidal tract lesion and rigidity from Parkinsonian syndrome.

Wartenberg wheel
A wheel with pins attached to it. It is used for testing dermatomal sensation by rolling the wheel and the pins across the skin (Fig. W.1).

Figure W.1: Wartenberg wheel

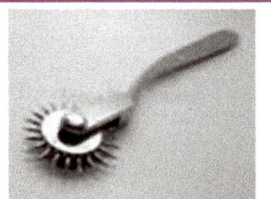

Wartenberg's sign
A sign of ulnar neuropathy where the patient is asked to place the forearm fully pronated on a table and then instructed to extend all the fingers. Then the patient is asked to abduct all the fingers, and then, adduct all of them. In ulnar nerve pathology, the little finger lags behind due to the weakness of extensor digiti minimi.

Wartenberg's syndrome
Mononeuropathy following entrapment of superficial branch of radial nerve. It is characterized by numbness, tingling and weakness of the posterior region of the thumb. It is also known as *cheiralgia paresthetica*.

Wartenberg's thumb adduction sign
An associated movement of the thumb that occurs

with forcible finger flexion in corticospinal tract lesion and has been equated with the Babinski reflex in the lower limb. The movement consists of adduction, flexion, and opposition of the thumb following active flexion of the terminal phalanges of the four fingers by the examiner and the patient hooking his fingertips and pulling with both hands. Normally, the thumb remains in abduction and extension.

Warwick's oculomotor nucleus complex The nucleus of the oculomotor nerve is not a single one but it is broken into a number of smaller complexes, each one supplying a specific extraocular muscle of the eye. Thus the anterior group has two nuclei, anteromedial and an anterolateral group, while the posterior one has six subsets five of which are symmetrical and are in both the sides of the midbrain and the sixth one is central, supplying both the eyes. This central nucleus supplies the levator palpebrae superioris and thus a lesion here causes mild ptosis in both the eyes. The Edinger–Westphal nucleus is located nearby and it sends sympathetic fibers to the pupillary muscles.

Wassermann test An antibody test for syphilis, based on complement fixation and it was the first hematological test for the disease. Blood or cerebrospinal fluid is admixed with the antigen, cardiolipin, extracted from bovine heart and nonspecific syphilis antibodies react with cardiolipin. However, it is not a specific test and can be positive in systemic lupus erythematosus, tuberculosis or malaria. Recently, in young stroke, APLA antibodies can also be detected by this test. This test is not much reliable for the diagnosis of primary syphilis, since sufficient antigen is not produced.

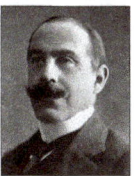

August von Wassermann (1866–1925, Germany)

Waterhouse–Friderichsen syndrome A complication of meningococcal meningitis where there is bleeding into the adrenal gland leading to its failure. The clinical features include organ failure, coma, hypotension, disseminated intravascular coagulation with purpuric spots, shock and eventual death. Treatment consists in immediate infusion with intravenous corticosteroids and antibiotics.

Weber test A clinical test to detect conductive deafness. A vibrating tuning fork is placed on the vertex of the patient and he or she is asked to indicate in which ear does it sound more. In conductive deafness, the sound is lateralized to the affected side. In sensorineural deafness it is better heard with the normal ear.

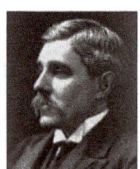

Frederick Parkes Weber (1863–1962, United Kingdom)

Weber's syndrome A variety of crossed hemiplegia where there is oculomotor nerve palsy with contralateral hemiplegia. The lesion is usually a vascular one in the midbrain. It is to be remembered that he did not describe conditions like Sturge–Weber syndrome, Klippel–Trénaunay–Weber syndrome or Osler–Rendu–Weber syndrome. These were described by his son. Incidentally, Weber was a dermatologist who described many conditions pertaining to skin diseases.

Webster Scale A clinical scale to assess the severity of Parkinson's disease. It consists of 10 items namely, tremor, rigidity, bradykinesia, postural instability, loss of arm swing, gait, facies, voice, seborrhea and activity of daily living. Each item is assigned a value, ranging from 0 to 3 in increasing order of severity. Thus the patient with the highest severity will score 30.

Weigert's law Destruction of tissue results in compensatory replacement and overproduction of new tissue during the process of regeneration or repair or both.

Weigert's stain This stain is used for nerve tissue with potassium dichromate to preserve myelin lipids. The lipids are then stained with the use of hematoxylin, and the pathways appear black due to the staining of myelin sheaths.

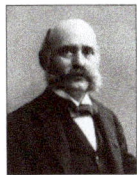

**Karl Weigert
(1845–1904, Germany)**

Werdnig–Hoffmann syndrome A recessively inherited disease manifesting in infancy at about 6 months of age. There is hypotonia, proximal weakness, fasciculations, kyphoscoliosis etc. The mother gives the history of less fetal movement in the third trimester, as in Zellweger syndrome. The prognosis is fatal.

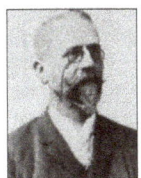

**Guido Werdnig
(1844–1919, Germany)**

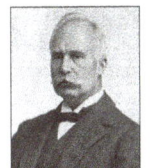

**Johann Hoffmann
(1857–1919, Germany)**

Wernicke's aphasia Also known as receptive, sensory or posterior aphasia, there is difficulty in comprehension of spoken or written language. The speech is fluent, non-sensical, paraphasic and replete with jargons, knight's move, where the subjects drifts from a topic to another, like the movement of the knight in the chess board, and neologisms, while retrieval of words is poor. They are typically unaware of their ailment and have little insight into the gravity of their problem. It is commonly caused by occlusion of the left middle cerebral artery in lesion of the posterior superior temporal gyrus.

Wernicke's area It refers to Brodmann area 22 located in the posterior part of the left or dominant superior temporal gyrus. It is concerned with the comprehension of written or spoken language. Lesion in this area leads to fluent aphasia which is fast and nonsensical and that is the reason it is often called jargon aphasia.

Wernicke's cramp A rare form of localized muscle cramp precipitated by movement.

Wernicke's encephalopathy A disorder of the central nervous system caused by depletion of thiamine or vitamin B1 from the body. It forms a component of *Korsakoff's syndrome* and if they occur simultaneously, the condition is known as *Wernicke–Korsakoff syndrome*. It is characterized by the triad of ophthalmoplegia, mostly affecting the lateral rectus muscle, ataxia and confusional state though all patients do not display all the three features. Other features include papilledema, pupillary changes, dysphagia, hearing loss, anterograde amnesia, psychosis, peripheral neuropathy, etc.

Since the condition is so often associated with involvement of other organs like, the heart and eyes, this condition is often referred to as *Wernicke's disease*. This condition is seen classically in alcohol abusers with malnutrition. Involvement of the tegmentum of the brain stem leads to pupillary changes, hypothalamic lesion leads to autonomic symptoms, medulla and cerebellum with ataxia, and anterior nucleus of thalamus and mammillary bodies with anterograde amnesia. The condition is treated with glucose infusion and thiamine injection with replenishment vitamin therapy and may even be reversible if consumption of alcohol is stopped.

Wernicke's hemianopic pupil In hemianopia, a reaction due to damage of the optic tract, consisting in loss of pupillary constriction when the light is directed to the blind side of the retina; pupillary constriction is maintained when light stimulates the normal side. This sign cannot be seen with a bright light because of intraocular scatter onto the seeing half of the retina.

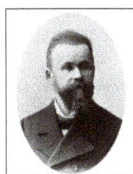

**Carl Wernicke
(1848–1905, Germany)**

Wernicke-Geschwind model of language An early neurological model for language devised by Wernicke that was later modified by Norman Geschwind.

Wernicke-Mann paralysis A form of hemiparesis with remarkable variability in the severity of involvement of the different muscle groups or the inequality of weakness in different muscle groups in a paretic limb during recovery.

West syndrome Also known as infantile spasms, this condition was described by William James West, a London practitioner, in his son in 1841 in a letter to *The Lancet* and Charles Bell examined the patient and in all likelihood, this is the only medical condition described by a father in his own offspring. It is a triad of infantile spasms, regression in milestones and a specific pattern in the EEG, known as hypsarrhythmia, a condition described by the eminent EEG expert Frederik Gibbs in 1952. In awake record, the background is chaotic and there are high amplitude, irregular spikes. It is seen in children between 3 and 12 months and myoclonic jerks, mostly in the flexor muscles, is the classical presentation and one such jerk is known as *Salaam attack*, as named by Charles Bell, where there is sudden flexion of the head and torso and bending of the hands which are drawn toward the chest. The disorder may be cryptogenic or secondary and the predisposing factors include tuberous sclerosis, cortical dysplasia, lissencephaly, Aicardi syndrome, microcephaly, Down syndrome, etc. Prednisolone, adrenocorticotropic hormone and vigabatrin are the useful drugs though the last named one may lead to loss of peripheral visual field. About half the number of the patients develop into Lennox–Gastaut syndrome.

Westphal's sign The other name for absent knee jerk. The jerk was originally described by Carl Westphal and Wilhelm Erb of Germany.

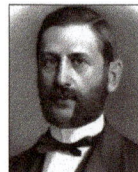

Carl Friedrich Otto Westphal (1833–1890, Germany)

Whytt's reflex Loss of pupillary reflex due to damage to the superior corpora quadrigemina.

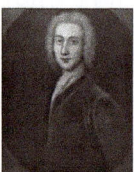

Robert Whytt (1714–1766, United Kingdom)

Wilbrand's knee The inferonasal fibers of the optic nerve enter the ipsilateral optic tract and then loop back to cross to the contralateral optic tract along with the ipsilateral superior temporal fibers. This is known as Wilbrand's knee. A lesion here causes junctional scotoma or *anterior chiasmal syndrome of Traquair*. A recent article stated that in primates, it is an artifact and the loop appears only after enucleation of an eye due to consequent loss of optic nerve fibers and the resultant shrinkage of the optic chiasma, which allows some fibers to enter the opposite optic tract.

Willis headache A variety of vascular headache following a stroke where the internal carotid artery is occluded. It is assumed that it is due to increased blood flow through the patent external carotid artery and the resultant pulsation.

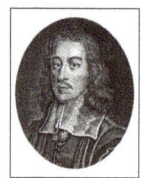

Thomas Willis (1621–1675, United Kingdom)

Willis' circle Described by Thomas Willis of England, it is an anastomotic circle in the base of the brain, consisting of anterior cerebral arteries, anterior communicating arteries, internal carotid arteries, posterior cerebral arteries and posterior communicating arteries of both sides. This is the site of aneurysms. The circle was described by Willis while he autopsied a subject whose one internal carotid artery was completely occluded, yet the subject never developed stroke. Willis felt that there must be some additional blood vessels in the brain which compensate for this block and supply the brain, and looking at the base of the brain he described the anastomotic circle.

Willis' paracusis The phenomenon of a deaf person hearing better in noisy surroundings.

Wilson's disease (please refer to any text book of neurology)

Wilson's pronator drift The other name for pronator sign where the patient is asked to hold both the arm horizontally in front with the palms upward. While closing the eye if the arms drift away it indicates loss of proprioceptive sense and the test is positive. This indicates mild muscular weakness from pyramidal tract lesion or choreiform disorder.

Wilson's pupil Eccentric pupil in neoencephalic diseases.

Wilson's sign Persistence of glabellar tap in Parkinson's disease.

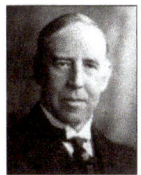

Samuel Alexander Kinnier Wilson (1878–1937, United Kingdom)

Wolfram syndrome The other name for DIDMOAD syndrome, the acronym meaning diabetes insipidus, diabetes mellitus, optic atrophy and deafness. It is inherited as an autosomal recessive condition.

Woltman's sign The other name for delayed or hung-up ankle jerk, found in hypothyroidism, type 2 diabetes mellitus or chronic propranolol therapy.

Wrisberg's nerve The other name for the nervous intermedius, a branch of facial nerve.

Wyburn-Mason syndrome A rare neurocutaneous syndrome characterized by arteriovenous malformations affecting the retina, visual pathways, midbrain and facial structures. It is usually unilateral and often asymptomatic. In some way it resembles Sturge–Weber syndrome though retinal malformations are not seen in the latter condition. It may manifest as torrential bleeding into the structures or chronic ischemia due to arteriovenous shunting of blood.

SECTION Y

Yim syndrome A congenital dysmorphic syndrome, presenting with severe skeletal and ocular involvement, macrocephaly, cortical atrophy, and hydrocephalus.

Yolken syndrome A congenital dysmorphic syndrome, characterized by genital and skeletal malformations, deafness, blindness and microcephaly.

Yom Kippur headache A variety of generalized constant headache in middle life, which happens during fasting. It is thought to be caused by dehydration and is relieved on lying down. For obvious reasons, persons belonging to the Muslim community experience it more during the Ramzan month.

Yoshimura reflex An alternate method of eliciting the extensor plantar response, where the middle of the sole is scratched and the great toe is extended.

Young syndrome A variety of hereditary motor neuropathy, which is dominantly inherited. It affects the arms before the legs and is often associated with laryngeal paralysis.

SECTION Z

Zellweger syndrome Also known as cerebrohepatorenal syndrome, it is a rare congenital disorder of autosomal recessive inheritance with absence of peroxisomes in the cells. Neuronal migration is impaired as is positioning and development. The patients are grossly hypotonic and often present with seizures and apnea. In the prenatal period, mothers may state that there is reduced fetal movement. There is reduction of cerebral myelin synthesis. Other features include hypoplastic supraorbital ridges, prominent epicanthal folds, hypoplastic midface and large fontanelle. Hepatomegaly in universal, as are renal cysts, punctuate calcification of cartilages. There is mutation in the genes that encode for peroxins, a protein required for the function of peroxisomes. There is accumulation of very long chain fatty acids and branched chain fatty acids since the peroxisomes are unable to degrade them.

Zimmerlin muscular dystrophy Hereditary muscular dystrophy with onset at the shoulder girdle.

Zinn's annulus A ring of fibrous tissue surrounding the optic nerve at the point of its entrance into the orbital apex. It divides superior orbital fissure into medial, central and lateral parts. The four extraocular recti muscles have origin from this ring. Important structures passing through the ring are superior division of oculomotor nerve, nasociliary branch of ophthalmic nerve, inferior division of the oculomotor nerve and the abducens nerve.

EU GSPR Authorised Reprsentative
Logos Europe, 9 rue Nicolas Poussin
1700, La Rochelle, France
Phone: +33 (0) 6 67 93 73 78
E-mail: contact@logoseurope.eu

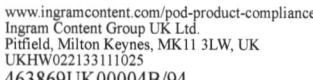

www.ingramcontent.com/pod-product-compliance
Ingram Content Group UK Ltd.
Pitfield, Milton Keynes, MK11 3LW, UK
UKHW022133111025
463869UK00004B/94